HAIRSTYLED

75 Ways to Braid, Pin & Accessorize Your Hair

ANNE THOUMIEUX

HAIRSTYLED

75 Ways to Braid, Pin & Accessorize Your Hair

Photographs by Brigitte Baudesson

Potter Style
New York

Published in the United States by Potter Style, an imprint of the Crown Publishing Group, a division of Penguin Random House LLC, New York.
www.crownpublishing.com
www.potterstyle.com

POTTER STYLE and colophon are registered trademarks of Penguin Random House LLC.

Originally published in French as *Coiffures Sur Mesure* by Hachette Livre (Marabout) in 2014.

Library of Congress Cataloging-in-Publication

Thoumieux, Anne.
[Coiffures sur mesure. English]
Hairstyled / Anne Thoumieux. — First Edition.
     pages cm
  Translation of: Coiffures sur mesure.
  1. Hairstyles. I. Title.
  TT972.T48613 2016
  646.7'24—dc23   2015017555

ISBN 978-0-553-45963-0
eBook ISBN 978-0-553-45973-9

Printed in China

Translated from the French by Nico LoVecchio

10 9 8 7 6 5 4 3 2

First US Edition

Contents

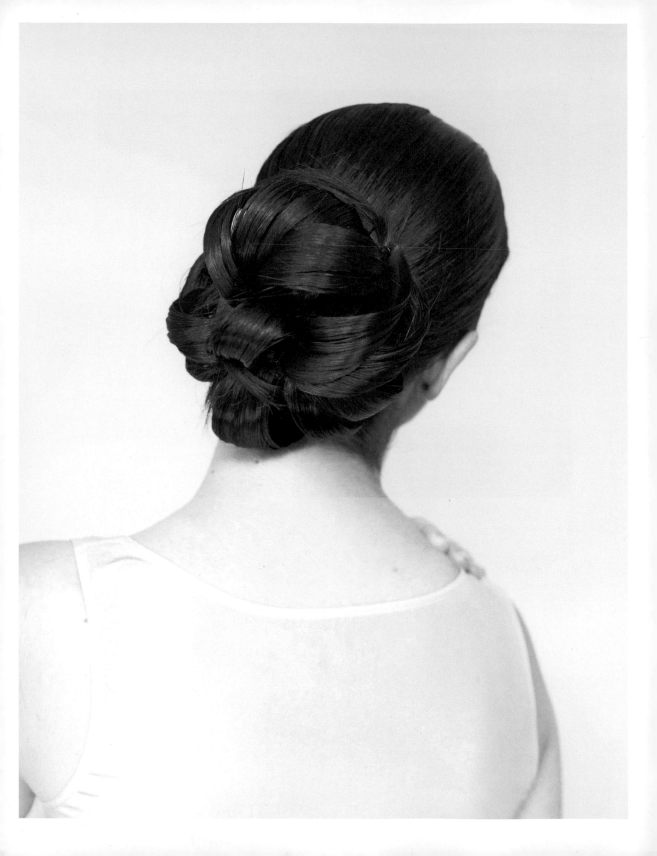

Doing Your Hair—
Easy as 1, 2, 3 …

There was a time when a proper lady wouldn't set foot outside without doing up her hair. Well, styling your hair is once again all the rage—but these days, we do it for fun! Who doesn't love to dress up their outfit with a simple braid, a sophisticated chignon, or beachy waves? Your hair is one of your best accessories, and you can upgrade your look with a few small steps. That's what this book is about: 75 step-by-step tutorials to give you lots of fresh ideas about how to upgrade your coif for all occasions, whether it be for everyday looks or special celebrations. These easy-to-master dos can be achieved with just a few simple steps. We've included plenty of helpful hints, plus a glossary of basic terms that might give you ideas for adding new products to your daily routine. So, ready for some no-fail hairstyling tips? Read on!

chapter 1

BUNS

in 9 styles

The Classic Bun · The French Twist
The Classic Chignon · The Chignon Twist · The Braided Chignon
The Braided Bun · The Bouffant Bun · The Flower Bun
The Bohemian Bun

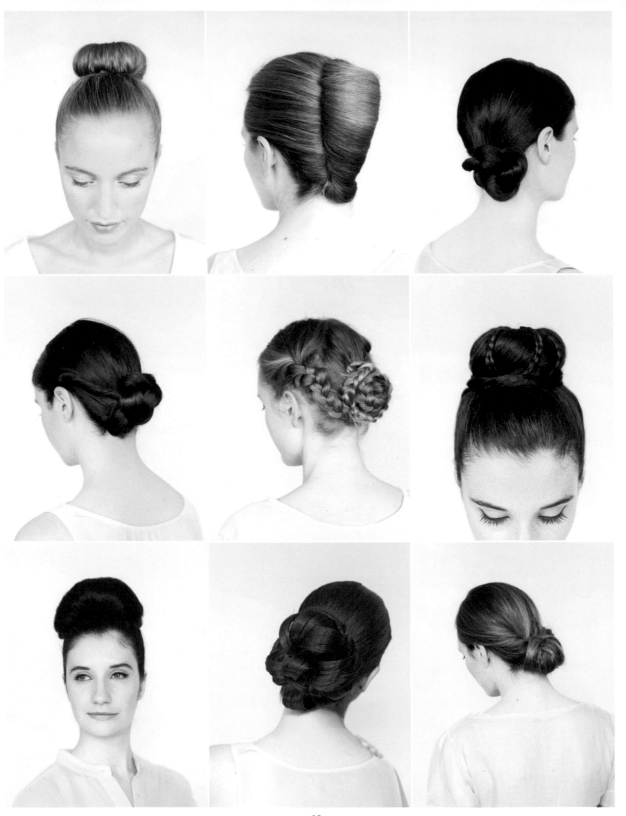

A must for any style repertoire, the bun is sure to lend an elegant feminine touch to your look, but is also suitable for the everyday. Whether you choose a simple style for the daily grind, or something more sophisticated for special occasions—for work, your best friend's wedding ... or even your own—you can't go wrong with a bun. Worn low or high, artsy or chic, messy or tight—the hard part is simply choosing. We'll leave that part up to you!

THE CLASSIC BUN

This classic ballerina-style bun worn high on the head is filled out using a foam ring hidden inside to add extra volume.

DIFFICULTY

YOU NEED
One foam hair donut, two hair elastics, fringe pins

TIP
If you have shorter hair, use some hair spray just before making your bun to improve hold, and then afterward to prevent flyaways.

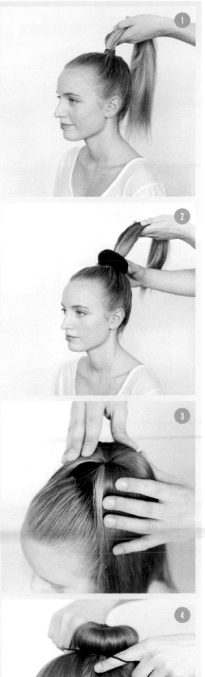

1 Make a high ponytail, securing with an elastic at the base.

2 Pull the ponytail through the center of the hair donut.

3 Spread your hair over the entire hair donut in order to hide it.

4 Place an elastic around the bun.

5 Wrap the remaining hair around the base of the bun underneath the hair donut and secure with fringe pins.

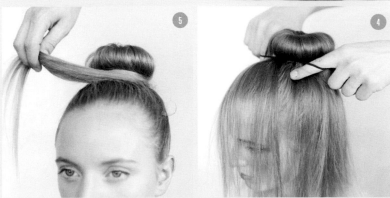

THE FRENCH TWIST

Using this simple method, wrapping your hair into a legendary French twist will be a cinch! Dress the twist up for a party or pair it with jeans and a plain T-shirt for a more casual look.

DIFFICULTY ХХХ

YOU NEED
A brush, bobby pins, fringe pins, one small clear elastic, hair spray

TIP
If you have shorter hair that tends to slip, place the elastic high up rather than toward the ends to make it easier to twist up your hair.

1 Brush all your hair to one side, then clip it into place in a vertical line using bobby pins. (You will flip your hair over this line in the next step.)

2 Attach the small elastic toward the ends of your hair, then flip the tied hair in the opposite direction as you brushed it to create a twist.

3 Conceal the end by folding it down into the bun, using your fingers to twist.

4 Tighten the twist as you tuck the remaining hair inward, then secure from top to bottom using fringe pins. Spritz with hair spray to set in place.

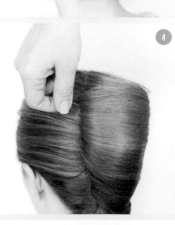

THE CLASSIC CHIGNON

This timeless feminine style will accentuate your neck and liven up your face in a flash. It's understated enough to pair with statement jewelry for a glitzy look.

DIFFICULTY

YOU NEED
A brush, two hair elastics, fringe pins, hair spray

TIP
Experiment with this style by varying the height of the ponytail or setting the chignon slightly askew.

1 Brush your hair and pull it into a low
   ponytail. Secure it with an elastic.

2 Separate the ponytail into two
   sections and twist the sections
   together, securing at the end with an
   elastic.

3 Wrap the twist back over itself and
   around the first elastic.

4 Secure the whole chignon in place
   with fringe pins and spritz with
   hair spray.

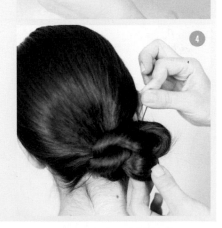

THE CHIGNON TWIST

A new twist on the classic chignon, this style incorporates a wide braided bun flanked by two twirled strands.

DIFFICULTY ✗ ✗ ✗

YOU NEED
A brush, two small clear elastics, fringe pins, hair spray

TIP

If you have very long hair, wrap the full braid several times through the small side twirls in order to conceal the elastic at the end.

1 Brush your hair, separate out two small sections, and twist them before bringing them together in a half ponytail. Secure with a small elastic.

2 Now separate your hair into three sections, incorporating the half ponytail into the center section.

3 Braid the sections as you would normally and finish with a small elastic at the end.

4 Flip the entire braid up and insert it back into the rest of your hair, between the two twirls, until you've achieved the desired chignon look.

5 Secure with fringe pins and spritz with hair spray.

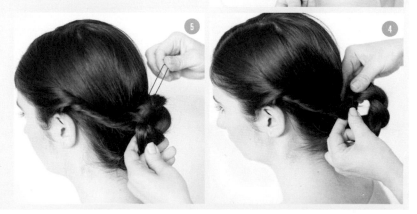

THE BRAIDED CHIGNON

Several strands weave together to form one big beautiful braided chignon. Subtle from the front, this intricate style will impress from the back.

DIFFICULTY ✗ ✗ ✗

YOU NEED
A brush, three small clear elastics, fringe pins, hair spray

TIP
To add volume to this style, divide the middle section into two separate braids, or use clip-in hair extensions.

1 Brush your hair into three separate sections. Braid the left section starting from the temple and secure with a small elastic.

2 Braid the right section starting from the right temple and secure with an elastic.

3 Braid the remaining center section and secure with an elastic.

4 Wrap the central braid over itself into a bun and secure with fringe pins, then crisscross the two side braids underneath.

5 Wrap the side braids around the central braided bun, secure with fringe pins, and tuck the ends under to conceal. Spritz with hair spray.

THE BRAIDED BUN

A simple bun has its place, but this glamorous braided version is a twist on the legendary style.

DIFFICULTY

YOU NEED
One foam hair donut, one hair elastic, several small clear elastics, fringe pins

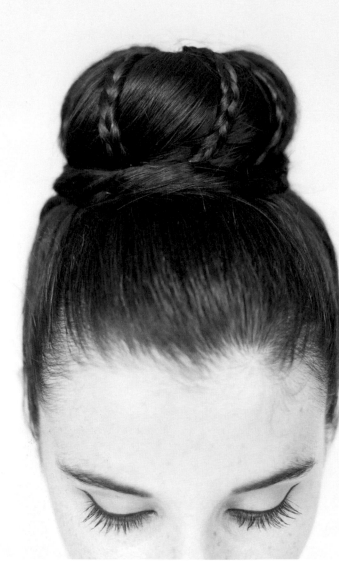

TIP

Depending on the length of your hair, wrap the final section of hair either forward or backward to conceal the ends.

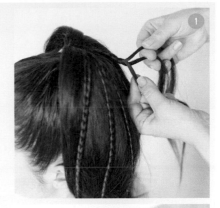

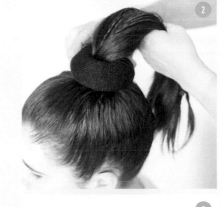

1 Make a ponytail high on your head and braid six or seven small bunches of hair out of this ponytail, securing each with a small elastic.

2 Pull the ponytail, including the braided portions, through the center of the hair donut.

3 Spread your hair the entire way around the hair donut in order to hide it, and space out the small braids over the bun.

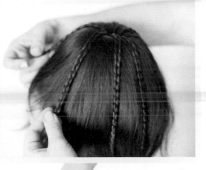

4 Pull the hair elastic around the whole bun and secure underneath.

5 Wrap the remaining length of hair around the base of the bun and secure with fringe pins.

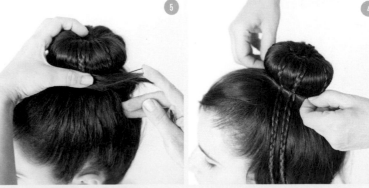

THE BOUFFANT BUN

This elegant, flowing updo is almost an accessory in itself.

DIFFICULTY ✂✂✂

YOU NEED
Two hair elastics, fringe pins, hair spray

TIP
If you have fine or unruly hair, using hair spray, hair gel, or fixing mousse to texturize it will help stabilize the bouffant.

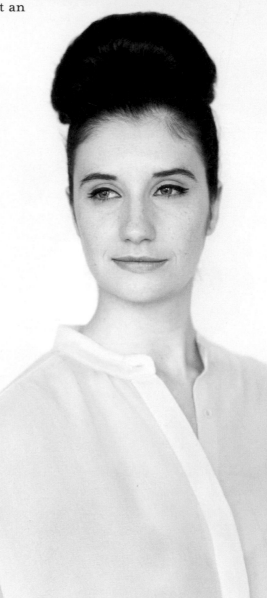

1 Make a ponytail high on your head, using a hair elastic at the beginning and toward the end.

2 Flip the length of hair toward the front to create a sort of pouf.

3 Sticking your fingers underneath the first elastic closer to your head, grab the elastic holding the other end, and pull underneath.

4 Wrap the remaining length of hair around the first elastic to conceal it, securing with fringe pins. (This will be visible from the back.)

5 Fan out the pouf portion left and right, secure with fringe pins, and spritz with hair spray.

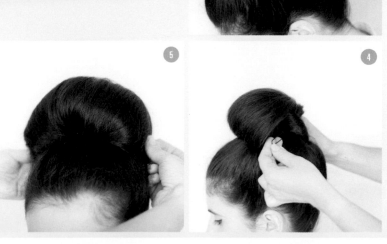

THE FLOWER BUN

A bridal-inspired look, this stunning bun will suit the most sophisticated of soirees!

DIFFICULTY ✕ ✕ ✕

YOU NEED
A brush, a hair straightener, one hair elastic, bobby pins, fringe pins, hair gel, hair spray

TIP
If your hair slips out of place, put small clear elastics at the end of each lock of hair, making it easier to pass through the large elastic without slipping.

26

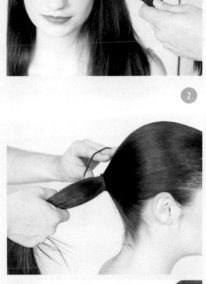

1 Brush your hair and straighten it with a hair straightener.

2 Pull your hair back into a ponytail and secure loosely with an elastic.

3 Using your fingers, flatten out a lock with some gel and make a curl shape.

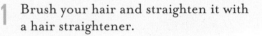

4 Stick the end of the lock into the elastic and secure against your head using a bobby pin. Repeat this process for the rest of the hair in the ponytail, creating flower petal shapes out of each lock.

5 Reinforce the bun using fringe pins and spritz with hair spray.

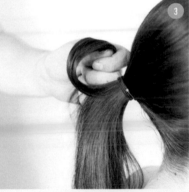

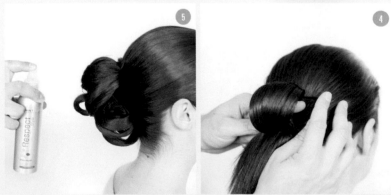

THE BOHEMIAN BUN

This romantic bun's intertwining twirls
lend it a free-spirited look.

DIFFICULTY ✗ ✗ ✗

YOU NEED
One hair elastic, two small clear
elastics, fringe pins, texturizing spray
or powder

TIP
*If your hair is long enough
and you want a messier look,
tease some strands and pull them
through the center section
several times.*

1 Spray texturizing spray or powder over your hair to make the strands stick together. Then, using your fingers, make a low ponytail and separate it into two sections above the elastic.

2 Pull the length of hair over and through the partition, allowing a twist to form on each side.

3 Make small braids or twists with the remaining hair, securing them with small elastics.

4 Pull all these through the center and arrange to your liking, securing them to the two initial twists using fringe pins.

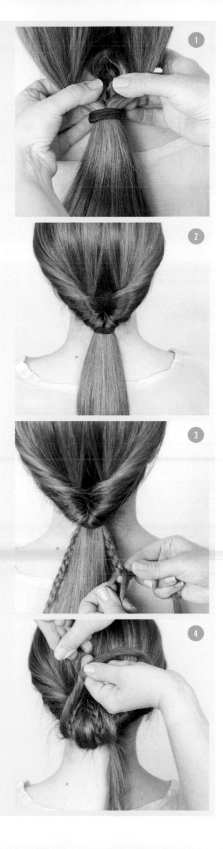

chapter 2

BRAIDS

in 9 styles

The Fishtail · The French Braid
The Four-Strand Braid · The Basic Crown
The Woven Crown · The Fishtail Crown · The Double Braids
Hippie Tresses · The Princess Plait

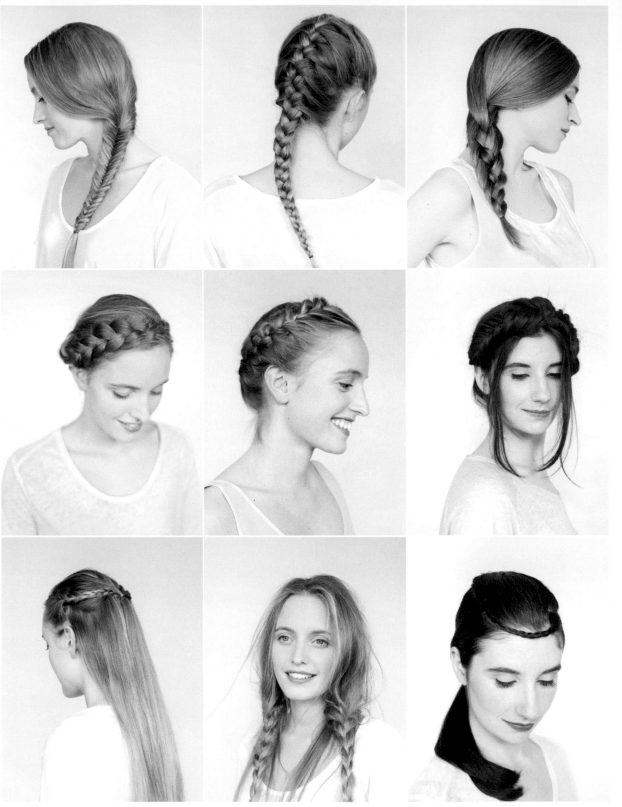

Whether you want a casual, chic, or classic look, the possibilities are endless with braids. An in-vogue, versatile choice for various lengths of hair, braids can be a miraculous tool for tailoring your look and giving your hair some extra personality. Once you've learned the basic braids, mastering more creative styles will be a breeze. Get those fingers working!

THE FISHTAIL

This elegant braid tightly blends four
strands of hair together rather than the
traditional three.

DIFFICULTY ✂ ✂ ✂

YOU NEED
A brush, one small clear elastic,
one hair elastic, scissors

TIP
*If your hair is layered
or damaged, blend shorter
sections in with longer sections
in order to keep the ends from
sticking out.*

1. Brush out any tangles in your hair, or straighten it if you have curly hair. Make a low ponytail and secure with the small clear elastic, then separate the ponytail into two equal parts. Grab a section with each hand.

2. Pull out a small section from the outside portion of each of the two main sections, and cross these over each other so the sections end up on the opposite side from where they started.

3. Starting once again with two main sections, repeat the process for the remaining length of hair, crisscrossing a small section from the outside of each main section over to the main section opposite, tightening the braid as you go.

4. The braid will take on the fishbone shape as each layer builds upon the last. Secure at the end with the hair elastic.

5. Cut off the small clear elastic at the top and gently massage the braid to relax it.

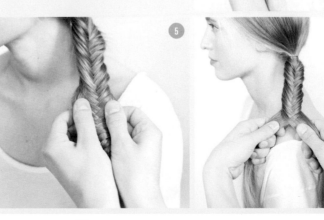

THE FRENCH BRAID

This takeoff on the basic braid offers so many styling possibilities and instantly makes you look put together.

DIFFICULTY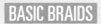

YOU NEED
One hair elastic

TIP

Each time you crisscross a section of hair, make sure you tighten up the braid to that point. If any section is too loose, it could stick out from the rest.

1   Pull out a medium-size section of
hair from the top of your head,
separate it into three sections, and
make two standard braids.

2   Now, as you cross one section over to
the other side, this time incorporate
a section of hair from the remaining
hair on the side of your head.

3   Repeat the process on the other side.
Then continue alternating between
left and right, adding in a section
of free hair from each side as you
go along.

4   Once all hair from the sides has been
woven into the braid, finish braiding
as you would normally and secure
with a hair elastic.

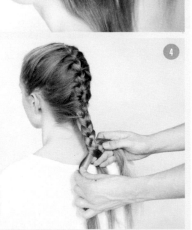

THE FOUR-STRAND BRAID

This unique, classy braid recalls days of yore. By pulling it over to one side, this style shows off the extra strand that makes this braid unique.

DIFFICULTY ✗✗✗

YOU NEED
A brush, one hair elastic

TIP
Dampening or wetting your hair will make the braiding process easier, ensuring that each strand stays separate.

1 Brush your hair, then pull it to one side and separate it out into four sections at neck level, going from left to right.

2 Take the section closest to the front of your neck and weave it over the one next to it.

3 Then weave it underneath the following section.

4 Finally weave it above the last section.

5 Start the process over beginning with the section now closest to the front of your neck: over, under, and over again. Then repeat until the braid is complete and secure with a hair elastic.

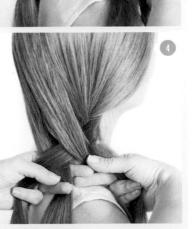

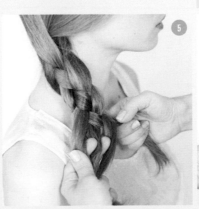

THE BASIC CROWN

This is the simplest crown to make, reserved for those with hair long enough to wrap the crown the whole way around.

DIFFICULTY ✗ ✗ ✗

YOU NEED
A brush, two small clear elastics, fringe pins, scissors

TIP
If you have medium-length hair, make a ponytail higher up, at ear level, in order to have enough hair to complete the crown.

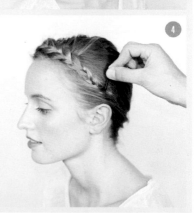

1 Brush your hair toward one ear, pull it into a ponytail and secure using a small elastic.

2 Braid the ponytail the whole way down, securing at the bottom with a small elastic. Cut off the elastic from the top.

3 Wrap the braid around your head, setting it in place with fringe pins as you go.

4 Conceal the end underneath your hair and secure with a fringe pin.

THE WOVEN CROWN

This romantic crown incorporates the French braid technique and is sure to turn heads.

DIFFICULTY ✂ ✂ ✂

YOU NEED
A brush, one small clear elastic, fringe pins

TIP
If you have short hair, use a hair extension matching your hair color, braid it, and set it around your real hair pulled back into a bun.

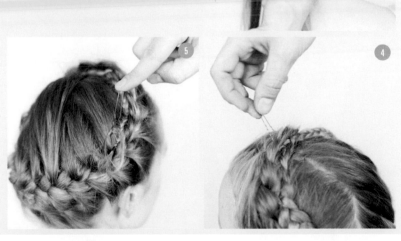

1 After brushing, separate out a third of your hair at the front and start by making a French Braid (page 36). This braid will extend from one ear, across the front, and then to the back of your head.

2 Continue all the way around, incorporating hair into the braid from the surrounding remaining hair.

3 Once you've reached the back, pull sections of hair alternately from below, toward the nape, and from above, toward the crown.

4 Secure with a small elastic and conceal it underneath the braid.

5 Stabilize the crown all around using fringe pins.

THE FISHTAIL CROWN

Bringing together two majestic braids and stray strands at your whim, this crown is a fresh take that will intrigue those around you.

DIFFICULTY ✕ ✕ ✕

YOU NEED
A brush, several small clear elastics, fringe pins

TIP

For a more natural look, loosen up the weaves of the braid once it is complete, or even let some strands fall out from underneath the crown.

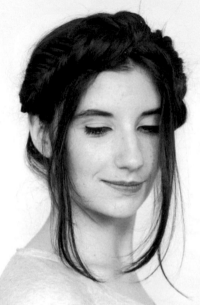

1 After brushing, part your hair at the
top and separate it into two equal
parts. Attach a small elastic to each
section above the ear, keeping some
strands in the front loose if you like.

2 Braid one side into a Fishtail
(page 34).

3 Secure the braid with a small elastic
and fix it atop your forehead with
fringe pins.

4 Repeat this process for the opposite
side, concealing the elastic end
underneath the opposite braid.

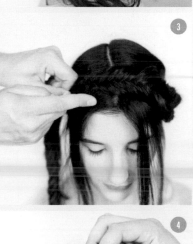

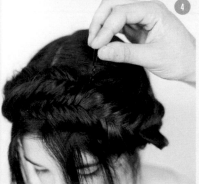

THE DOUBLE BRAIDS

Two simple braids come together
at the back to create an enchantingly
simple style.

DIFFICULTY ✂ ✂ ✂

YOU NEED
A brush, three small clear elastics, scissors

TIP
*Vary the effect of this
style by braiding each strand
entirely, or braiding only up
to where the various parts
come together.*

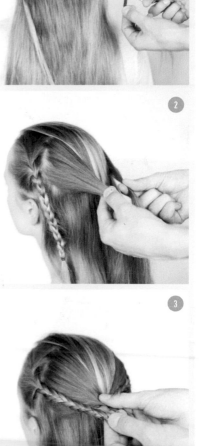

1 Brush your hair back. Pull out a
section of hair at the temple on each
side and braid each section toward
the back, securing with small elastics.

2 Pull out two sections of hair next to
these braids, straighten them out,
and hold them together at the back of
your head.

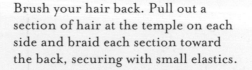

3 Bring the braids together just above
the straightened sections so that
each braid is overlapping the section
beneath it.

4 Secure all the parts in a half ponytail
using the third small elastic and cut
off the elastics from the individual
braids.

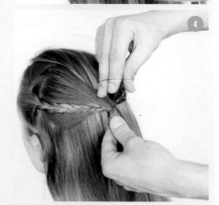

HIPPIE TRESSES

Here's a hip bohemian do that adds a touch of polish to a free-spirited look.

DIFFICULTY ✂ ✂ ✂

YOU NEED
A brush or a comb, two small clear elastics, texturizing powder

TIP
If your hair slips out of place, use some hair gel or fixing mousse as you begin braiding to make sure the braids set well. Finish off with elastics.

1 Part your hair in the center, then apply some texturizing powder to the roots and along the lengths of the hair.

2 With a brush or comb, lightly tease the first third of the hair starting at the roots. (This will help prevent the braids from coming undone.)

3 Braid the remaining lengths of hair, making the braids tighter as you go along.

4 Heavily tease the ends to finish off the braid, or secure each braid with a small clear elastic. Pull out some stray strands for effect and spritz with hair spray.

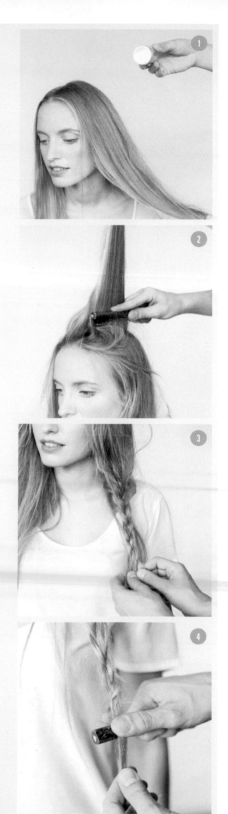

THE PRINCESS PLAIT

This chic but sharp style will highlight your forehead and neck.

DIFFICULTY ✗ ✗ ✗

YOU NEED
One hair elastic, one small clear elastic, hair gel or fixing mousse

TIP

For the experts out there, try incorporating a French Braid (page 36) where the braid meets up with the part, or make a mini braid for an even more unique effect.

1 Separate out a small section of hair from the left or right side of your forehead.

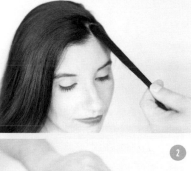

2 Pull back a good amount of hair from the forehead, coat it with gel or mousse, and smooth it out as you pull it toward the back of your head.

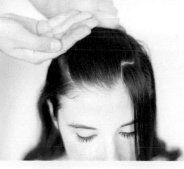

3 Braid or twist this hair.

4 Pull it into a ponytail at the base of your neck, using the hair elastic to secure it to the rest of your hair.

5 Braid the small front section and secure with the small elastic. Then pull this braid across your forehead and align it with the part on the opposite side, blend it in with the rest of your hair, and secure it with a hidden pin.

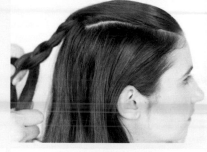

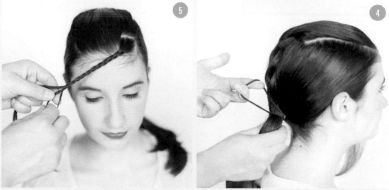

chapter 3

HEADBANDS

in 6 styles

————————————

The Asymmetric Headband · The Hip Headband
The Classic Headband · The Regal Headband
The Pouf · The Headband Bun

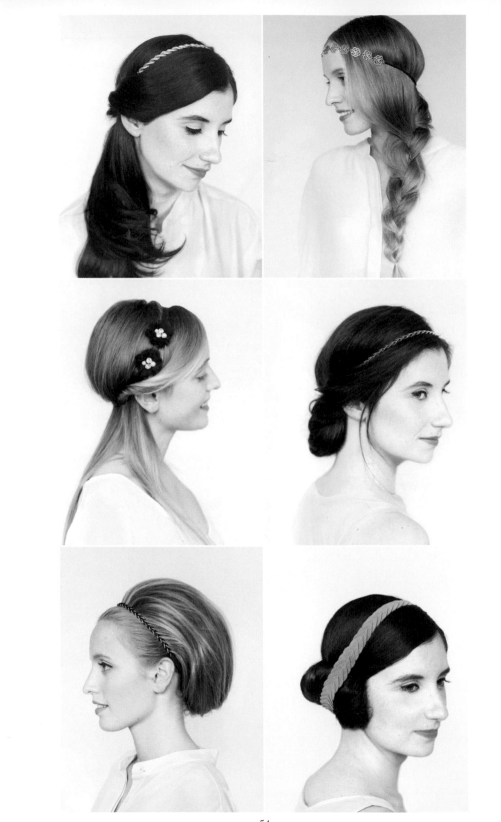

More than just a functional piece to hold your hair back, headbands are a fashionable way to add some extra flair to your hair. Traditionally considered a casual accessory, headbands can now dress up even the most sophisticated of hairstyles. We'll show you how to make the most of this versatile accessory, whether for a relaxed everyday look or a night on the town.

THE ASYMMETRIC HEADBAND

A dramatic sweep of hair over one shoulder offsets a poised headband in this regal style. For a more casual look, try a dressed-down headband, such as something with florals or denim.

DIFFICULTY ✕ ✕ ✕

YOU NEED
A brush, a headband, one small clear elastic

TIP
To emphasize the asymmetry, you can pull some strands into a ponytail or a bun on the side.

1 Brush your hair to one side and
drape it over your shoulder.

2 Place the headband on your head,
extending backward from the crown
to the nape of the neck. Pull a small
section from the front side opposite
the shoulder over which you've
draped your hair and tuck it under
the headband.

3 Pull a small section over from the
shoulder side and wrap it around the
headband. Then continue alternating
this process side to side.

4 Arrange the various sections so they
cover the side of the headband, and
secure on the side with a small elastic.

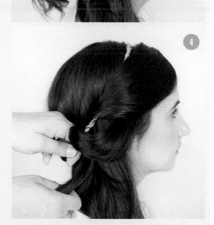

THE HIP HEADBAND

Grab your favorite headband and sport this casual but on-trend look. This style works best with a fairly flat headband that will hold its place.

DIFFICULTY ✂ ✂ ✂

YOU NEED
A brush, a headband, one hair elastic

TIP
Vary the technique used—two braids, no braid, twists …

1   Part your hair in the middle and brush both sides.

2   Arrange each section of hair over your ears, then pull both sides together and drape over one shoulder.

3   Put on the headband, setting it high up on the forehead.

4   Weave the lower section into a loose, slightly messy braid and secure with an elastic.

THE CLASSIC HEADBAND

This understated style will gracefully hold your hair in place.

DIFFICULTY ✂ ✂ ✂

YOU NEED
A brush, a narrow headband

TIP
If the headband tends to hike up on your head, use a tighter (but still flexible) one, and secure your hair using bobby pins.

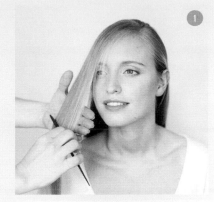

1 Part your hair on one side and brush both sides, leaving a section free at the front.

2 Place the headband high on your head, covering all your hair, and set firmly at the nape below.

3 Free up the section at the front and pull it down toward your ear.

4 Twist as you insert this hair into the headband at the back.

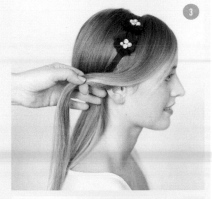

THE REGAL HEADBAND

Here's an easy but elegant winner for both day and night, which also works well with bangs.

DIFFICULTY ✗ ✗ ✗

YOU NEED
A headband, one small clear elastic, fringe pins

TIP
Tilt your head forward as you put on the headband. This will help situate the headband correctly at the nape of your neck, preventing it from hiking up later.

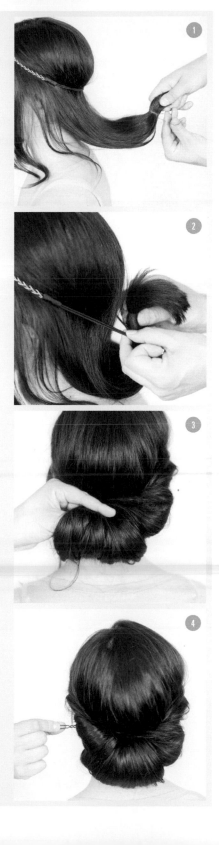

1 Part your hair in the middle or on the side, then place the headband on your head, covering your hair at the nape of your neck and at the desired height in the front. You won't move the headband after this step, so take care to put it exactly where you'd like it. Drape your hair over your back and secure with a small elastic an inch or two above the ends.

2 Bring the elastic up over the headband.

3 Roll the hanging bunch of hair up over itself, tucking it in around the headband.

4 Even out the bun formed and secure with fringe pins.

THE POUF

A bouffant updo along with a classy headband make this style fit for an edgy First Lady.

DIFFICULTY ✗ ✗ ✗

YOU NEED
A comb, a headband, fringe pins, hair spray

TIP
For a classier effect, pull out two wide sections of hair from each side at the front and insert these into the band of hair last, over the headband, so that only an inch or two of the front of the headband is visible.

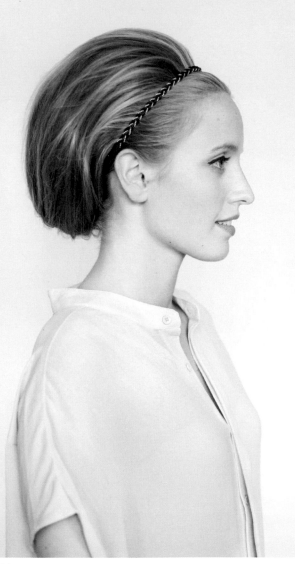

1 With the headband around your neck, use a comb to tease all your hair, starting at the roots and going up about halfway.

2 Once you've worked up a thick mass of hair, pull the headband up over your face and set it in place.

3 Twist the ends of your hair together without flattening out the teased effect.

4 Tuck the twisted ends underneath the headband at nape level.

5 Set with fringe pins and spritz with hair spray.

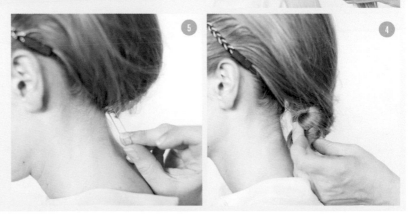

THE HEADBAND BUN

A stylish headband graces a slightly
off-center chignon for a
retro-meets-modern look.

DIFFICULTY ✂ ✂ ✂

YOU NEED
A wide, flexible headband, one hair elastic,
fringe pins

TIP
*This style can also be done
with a braid or a messy
chignon. Use hair spray for
better hold.*

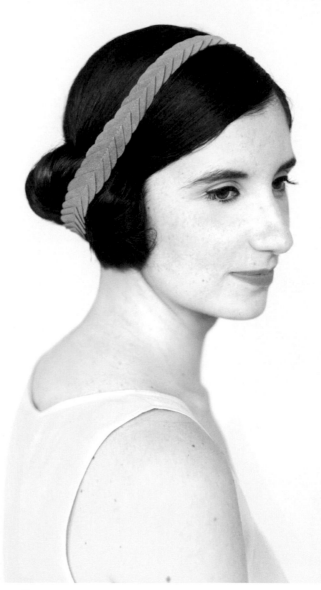

1 With the headband around your neck, pull your hair to one side and set it in a low ponytail at ear level, securing it with an elastic.

2 Twist the ponytail over on itself into a bun.

3 Secure the bun with fringe pins.

4 Place the headband around your head, with the bottom at nape level and around the bun to hold it in place.

chapter 4

ACCESSORIES

in 9 styles

Dressy Barrettes • Fashion Barrettes
Half-Ponytail Barrettes • The Stylish Comb
Scattered Flowers • The Crisscross Ribbon • The Pirate
The Headband • The Scarf Bow

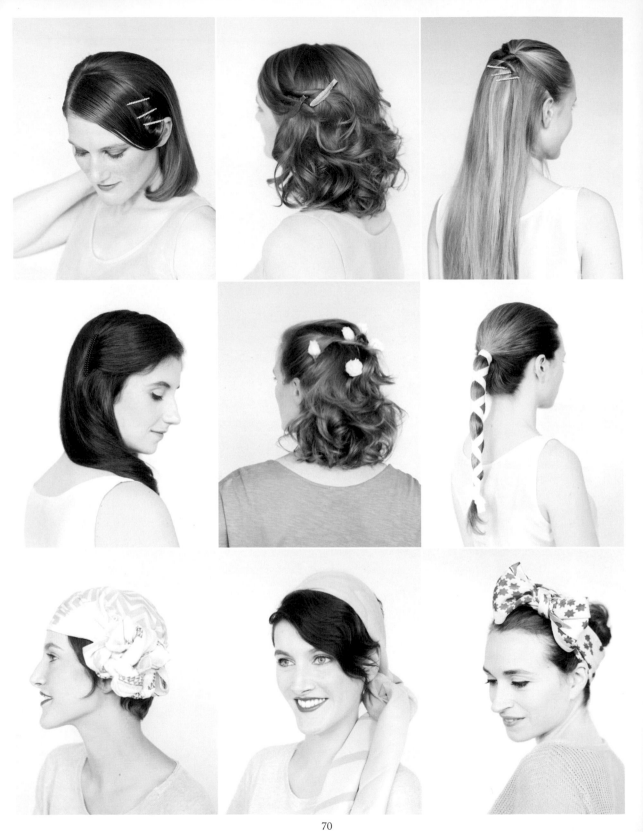

Sometimes, a hairstyle is more about the accessories than about the actual do. You know, those times when you just can't pass up those cute barrettes, that classy clip, that beautiful scarf . . . Maybe some glitz, glam, even a little bling to surprise your friends? The accessories in this chapter can also be used with any of the other styles in the book—feel free to get creative and mix things up!

DRESSY BARRETTES

A touch of belle époque class for all hair lengths.

DIFFICULTY ✗ ✗ ✗

YOU NEED
A comb, several fairly long flat barrettes, styling mousse, hair spray.

TIP
Choose different barrettes to adapt this style to any occasion—something simple for work, sparkly for a night out, or loud for a vacation.

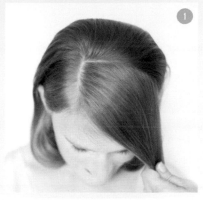

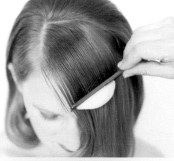

1 Part your hair to one side, then straighten and separate out a section in the front.

2 Apply some mousse to this section and smooth using your fingers or a comb.

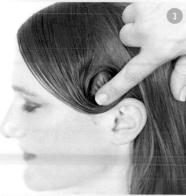

3 Roll this section up over itself to create a flat swirl.

4 Secure using barrettes, setting the first barrette across the twirl. Spritz with hair spray.

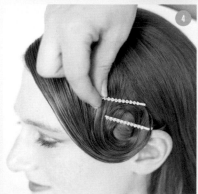

FASHION BARRETTES

This simple style is adaptable for all hair types, can be an everyday look, and is perfect when your hair is between lengths.

DIFFICULTY ✂ ✂ ✂

YOU NEED
A curling iron, several barrettes, hair spray

TIP
For a bohemian variation, choose small barrettes and set them among thin strands of hair.

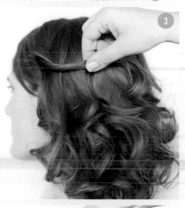

1 Curl your hair with a curling iron.

2 Spray with hair spray as you fluff using your fingers.

3 Pull out a small section from the front and twist back, setting it with a barrette on the side.

4 Repeat for a second small section. Feel free to add a third section and barrette.

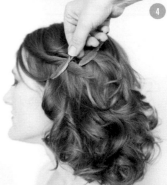

HALF-PONYTAIL BARRETTES

A classic gets jazzed up with an updated boho-chic look.

DIFFICULTY

YOU NEED
A brush, several flat barrettes

TIP
To create more volume, tease the top of the first section of hair and set the barrettes so as to puff up the hair.

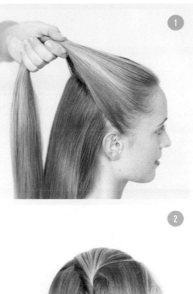

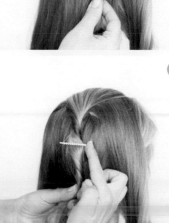

1 Brush your hair well to make sure there are no tangles, then pull it straight back.

2 Separate out a main section of hair, then twist.

3 Clip a barrette onto the twist.

4 Pull out another section of hair and twist, clipping another barrette onto the twist next to the first. Continue the process with as many barrettes as desired, keeping them flat on the back of the head.

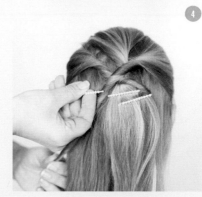

THE STYLISH COMB

Bring back a classic accessory with this
deceptively simple style.

DIFFICULTY ✗ ✗ ✗

YOU NEED
A brush, a decorative hair comb, straightening spray

TIP
*If your hair slips out of
place, spray some hair spray just
around the comb to stabilize it.
This will leave the rest of your
hair soft and flexible.*

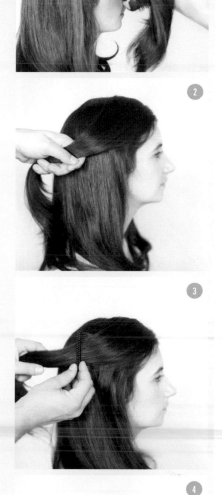

1 Brush your hair and spray with
   straightening spray.

2 Grab a section of hair on the side and
   pull it back.

3 Insert the hair comb with the teeth
   going toward your head, but the front
   of the comb facing toward your head.

4 Flip the comb back, then push it in
   firmly to fix the section in place.

SCATTERED FLOWERS

Add some springtime to your hair with this fun floral look. Feel free to use this method on other styles, such as braids and buns.

DIFFICULTY ✂ ✂ ✂

YOU NEED
Fresh flowers that will hold up (e.g., roses, baby's breath), a comb, one large alligator clip, fringe pins

TIP
To avoid damaging the petals, make sure the fringe pin goes through the firm center of the flower.

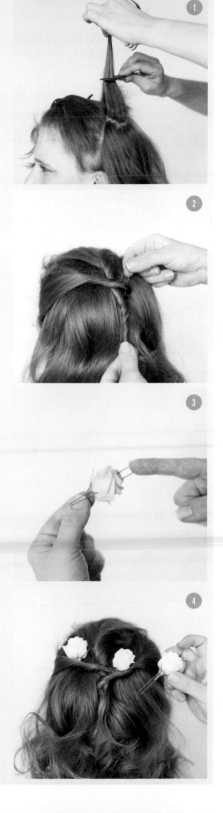

1 Clip the front half of your hair forward with the alligator clip, then use a comb to lightly tease the remaining hair on top in order to create a firm base.

2 Remove the hair clip and divide the front hair into three smaller strands. Twist each one and secure it with fringe pins to the base of the teased hair.

3 Stick a fringe pin through the center or stem of each flower.

4 Scatter the flower pins throughout your hair.

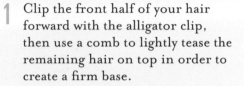

THE CRISSCROSS RIBBON

Here's a delightful way to liven up a simple ponytail.

DIFFICULTY ✂ ✂ ✂

YOU NEED

A long piece of ribbon, one hair elastic, one small clear elastic

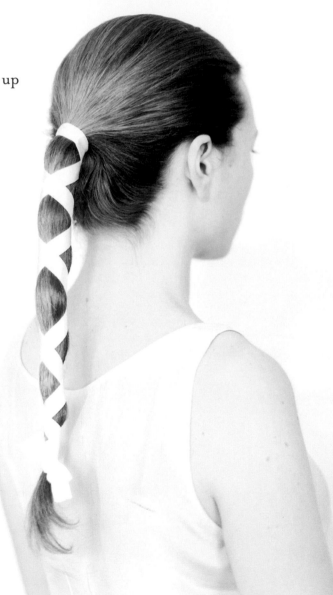

TIP

For a romantic bohemian effect, you can fasten some loose ribbons to the base of the ponytail.

1 Make a ponytail and secure it with a
hair elastic, then pass the middle of
the ribbon through the elastic and
wrap it once around the base of the
ponytail to hide the elastic.

2 Knot the ribbon underneath the
base, then crisscross the two lengths
of ribbon across the ponytail.

3 Continue crisscrossing the ribbon
the whole way down the ponytail.

4 Knot the ribbon at the bottom and
place the small elastic just below the
knot. Tie a bow with the ribbon on
top of the elastic to conceal it.

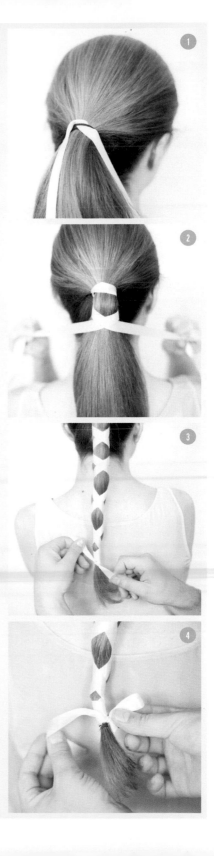

THE PIRATE

This style is music festival–ready. The scarf dresses up a simple outfit while keeping your head protected from the summer sun.

DIFFICULTY ✂ ✂ ✂

YOU NEED
A large square scarf, one bobby pin

TIP
Place the scarf over your forehead, not right at the hairline—direct contact with skin will prevent it from slipping.

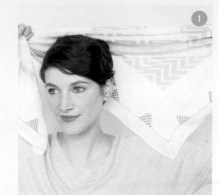

1 Fold the scarf into a triangle shape.

2 Place the base of the triangle at forehead level, putting pressure on the sides of your head as you pull the scarf back.

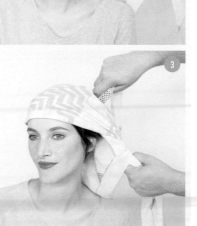

3 Make a large knot on the side using the edges of the scarf.

4 Tuck the point of the triangle underneath the knot and secure the scarf with a bobby pin.

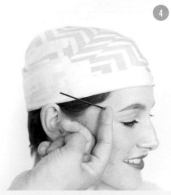

THE HEADBAND

This sporty style works great with any hairstyle and length—short, long, curly, straight, bangs—plus it's a quick and easy way to repurpose your scarf when you don't want to wear it anymore.

DIFFICULTY

YOU NEED
A large rectangular scarf, one bobby pin

TIP
The size of the scarf should be based on the length of your hair, so that the scarf ends are either shorter or longer than your hair.

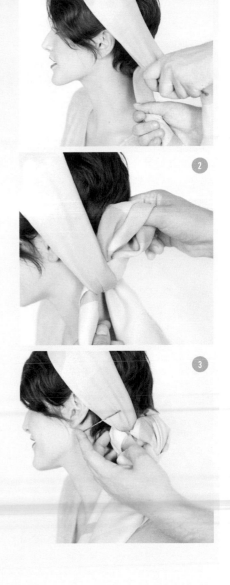

1 Fold or roll up the scarf to make it
   into a wide strip with the far edges in
   a point. Place it flat over your head,
   with your hair loose, and the two
   ends of the scarf toward the back.

2 Tie the two ends of the scarf at the
   lower back of your hair, slightly askew
   on the head.

3 Set with a bobby pin and drape the
   scarf ends forward over one shoulder.

THE SCARF BOW

Lots of pep plus a bit of vintage charm will liven up your look in seconds.

DIFFICULTY

YOU NEED
A fairly thin scarf, two bobby pins, fringe pins

TIP
If you have short or mid-length hair, forget about the bun and just let your hair down, or pull it into a ponytail.

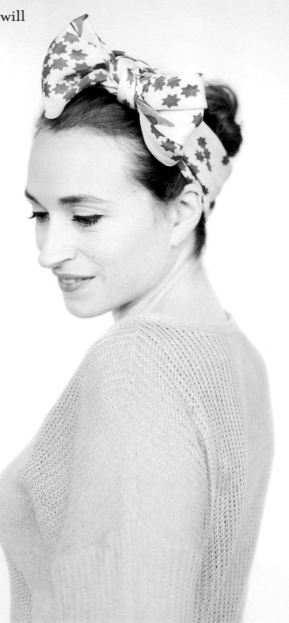

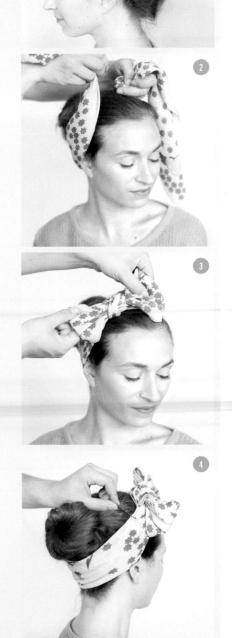

1   Pull your hair up into a quick bun and secure with fringe pins.

2   Fold the scarf lengthwise into a strip and place on the nape of your neck, holding an end of the scarf in each hand.

3   Pull the two ends forward and tie into a pretty, off-center bow.

4   Secure with bobby pins concealed behind the bow.

chapter 5

CURLY, WAVY, AND KINKY HAIR

in 9 styles

The Half Crown · Messy Curls · Crisscrossed Curls
The Masked Twist · The Shoulder Ponytail
The Twisted Crown · The Spiraled Braid
The Retro Pouf · The Punk's Pouf

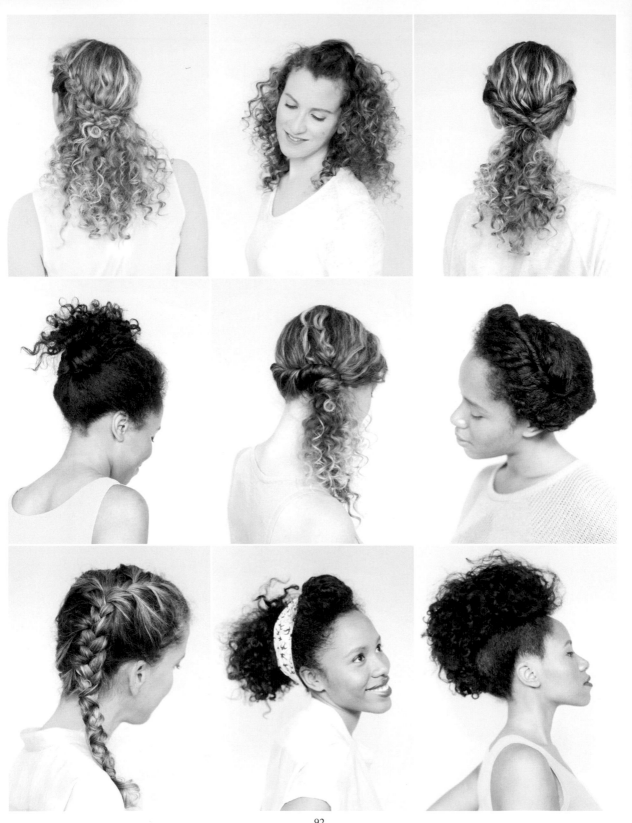

Though your ringlets look lovely on their own, sometimes you want an inventive style to do something different. Thankfully, it's not just our straight-haired friends who can whip up fabulous dos. *Au contraire,* those curls—or waves, or kinks—allow you to do things that straighter hair types can only dream of. Here we present our best ideas for not only taming those curls, but making the most of them!

THE HALF CROWN

Two pretty braids woven into hair worn loose will help keep those curls away from your face with style.

DIFFICULTY ⚔ ⚔ ⚔

YOU NEED
Two small clear elastics, fringe pins

TIP
If you have shorter or damaged hair, make two braids starting from the temples and attach them together to keep hair clear of your face.

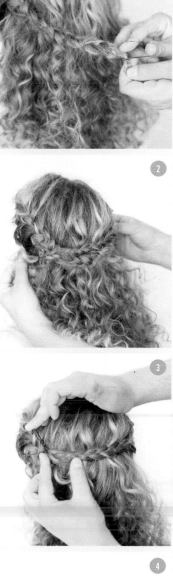

1   Part your hair in the middle, then braid a section on each side of your head, finishing each one with a small elastic.

2   Pull the two braids behind your head at the desired height, crisscrossing them horizontally.

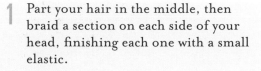

3   Secure them together using fringe pins.

4   Conceal the end of each braid under the start of the opposite braid and secure with a fringe pin.

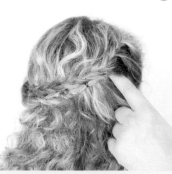

MESSY CURLS

You can spread this mass of curls out for maximum effect, or pull it together to open up your face.

DIFFICULTY ✂ ✂ ✂

YOU NEED
Several small clear elastics, one large alligator clip, bobby pins, fringe pins

TIP
For a trendier look, make twists all around your head, then pull them up into a high bun.

1 Take a good amount of hair from above your forehead and divide it into a few smaller sections.

2 Secure all sections but one with the alligator clip. Then twist the remaining free section and pull it back.

3 Secure the twisted section with a bobby pin, then repeat the process with the other sections of hair.

4 Intertwine the different sections and secure with fringe pins.

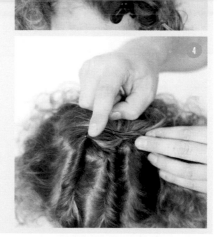

CRISSCROSSED CURLS

Here's a quick and easy style for every day!

DIFFICULTY ✗ ✗ ✗

YOU NEED
Bobby pins or fringe pins

TIP

To keep loose hair in place, make a low ponytail and crisscross the twists around the hair elastic.

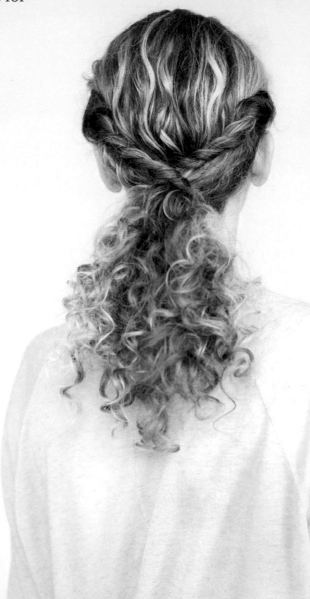

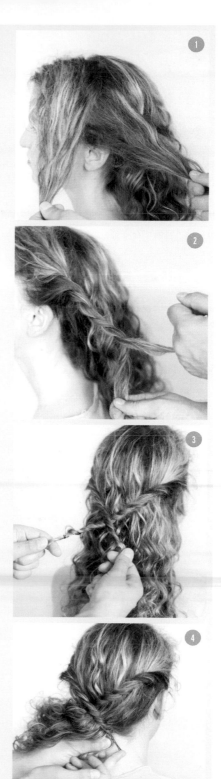

1 Pull out two small sections of hair on one side of your head.

2 Twist them together going from front to back.

3 Repeat this process with two sections of hair from the opposite side of your head. Then crisscross the two twists above the rest of your hair.

4 Now bring the twists over and around the rest of your hair so that they meet underneath at nape level and secure with bobby or fringe pins, depending on the thickness of the curls.

THE MASKED TWIST

This sassy variation on the French twist is designed especially to help tame frizz and can be worn every day!

DIFFICULTY ✗ ✗ ✗

YOU NEED
Fringe pins

TIP
If your hair is too short in front to reach the ponytail in the back, use a fringe pin to secure the shorter front sections so the hair doesn't hang loose.

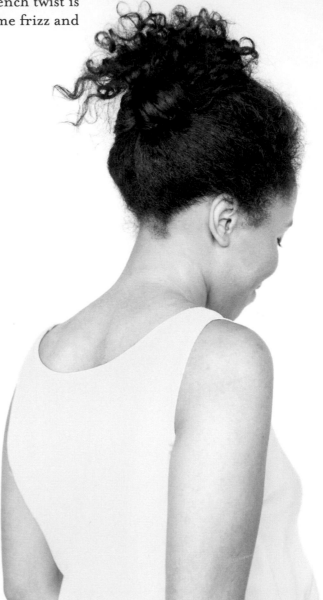

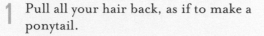

1 Pull all your hair back, as if to make a ponytail.

2 Twist the hair upward along its entire length.

3 Wrap the big twist over on itself without pulling it too tight, and secure with fringe pins.

4 Let the curly ends fall out toward the back and relax the twist with your fingers, letting some strands fall free.

THE SHOULDER PONYTAIL

This simple style is a unique way to tame your mane while subtly highlighting your neck.

DIFFICULTY ✂ ✂ ✂

YOU NEED
A comb, fringe pins

TIP
For a romantic look, untangle the curls over your shoulder, or even use a curling product to accentuate them.

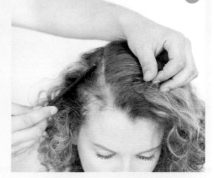

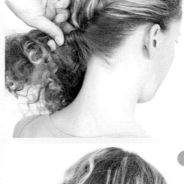

1 Part your hair on the side, then grab the lower portion.

2 Roll up this hair starting from the lower temple to create a twist, continuing toward the side opposite the part.

3 As you go along, secure above the nape with fringe pins.

4 Wrap the end of the twist around the free-hanging hair.

5 Secure from above with fringe pins and drape the rest over one shoulder.

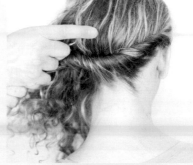

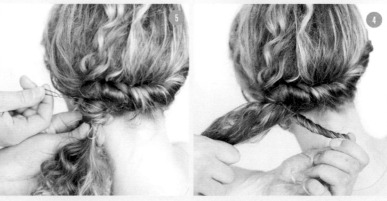

THE TWISTED CROWN

This fresh look highlights your face and neck and is a great style for when your hair feels frizzy.

DIFFICULTY 𝄤 𝄤 𝄤

YOU NEED
Bobby pins, fringe pins, two large alligator clips, straightening cream

TIP
Firmly tighten up the ends of the twists so they stand out against the rest of your hair and to prevent them from coming undone.

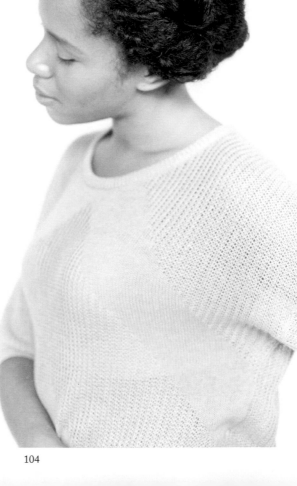

1 Divide your hair into three sections: one in front, one on the side, and one at the back. Use the alligator clips on the sections not being handled at each step.

2 Apply straightening cream to soften up the curls.

3 Twist the front section toward the back, above your ear, and fix at neck level with bobby pins.

4 Repeat the process with the side portion, going over your head, back, and parallel to the first. Secure firmly to your head with fringe pins.

5 Now pull all hair the together and twist further, across the back of your head at neck level, continuing in the same line as the other twists. Secure with fringe pins on the opposite side.

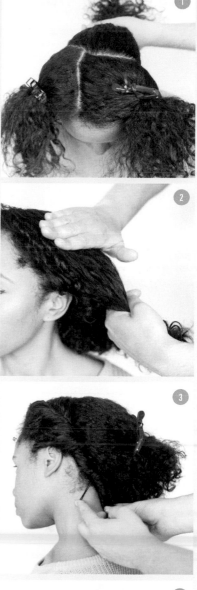

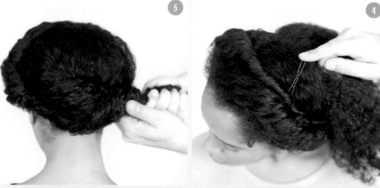

THE SPIRALED BRAID

This unique style plays up your curls by combining a simple braid with a spiraling strand.

DIFFICULTY ✗ ✗ ✗

YOU NEED
Two small clear elastics

TIP

For a rawer look, extend the spiral wrap all along the braid, incorporating random strands of hair from along the sides.

1   Work out any tangles in your hair, then begin a French Braid (page 36), using the front and side sections of hair.

2   Continue the braid to the end and secure with a small elastic, leaving the hair at neck level free.

3   Wrap that free section of hair around the braid in a haphazard pattern.

4   Attach the ends of the braid and the spiral together using a second small elastic.

THE RETRO POUF

A cheery style for every day, accentuated by a fun headband.

DIFFICULTY ✂ ✂ ✂

YOU NEED
An elasticized headband, one large alligator clip, bobby pins, one hair elastic

TIP
If you have curly rather than kinky hair, tease the main mass of hair for greater volume.

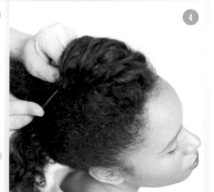

1 Pull out a triangle shape of hair from the top of your head and set it in place with the alligator clip.

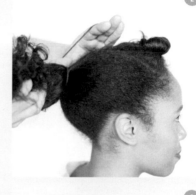

2 Pull the rest of your hair back into a high ponytail and secure with an elastic.

3 Unclip the triangle of hair, then twist it over on itself to create a pouf effect.

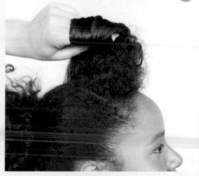

4 Secure at the edges with bobby pins.

5 Place the headband between the pouf and the ponytail.

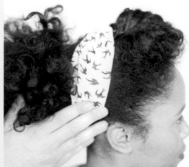

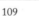

THE PUNK'S POUF

Sport this sassy, voluminous
do for a style that rocks!

DIFFICULTY ✗✗✗

YOU NEED
A brush, bobby pins, straightening cream

TIP
*To prevent the pouf from
slipping, make sure you really
bolster the sides with bobby
pins set in scattered rows.*

1   Using a brush and the straightening
    cream, straighten out your hair on
    one side moving upward.

2   Secure the stiff, untreated hair at the
    top using several bobby pins, half
    going from front to back and half
    going from back to front, all along
    the pouf in progress and ending at
    the nape of your neck.

3   Repeat this process on the other side,
    first applying straightening cream
    and pushing the hair up with the
    brush, then securing the stiff hairs
    high up with bobby pins.

4   Use your fingers to even out the hair
    forming the pouf and, if needed,
    even out the surface with the brush.

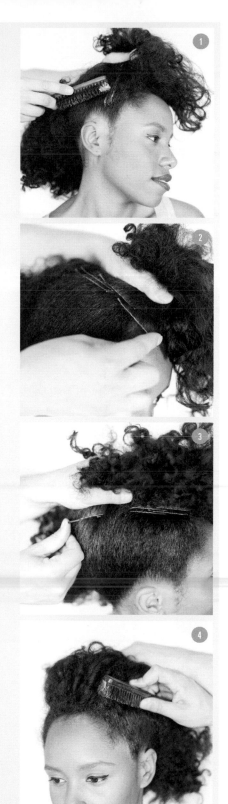

chapter 6

SHORT HAIR

in 6 styles

The Sleek Pixie · The New Wave
The Side Do · The Bedhead
The Pinned-Up Pouf · The Wavy Twenties

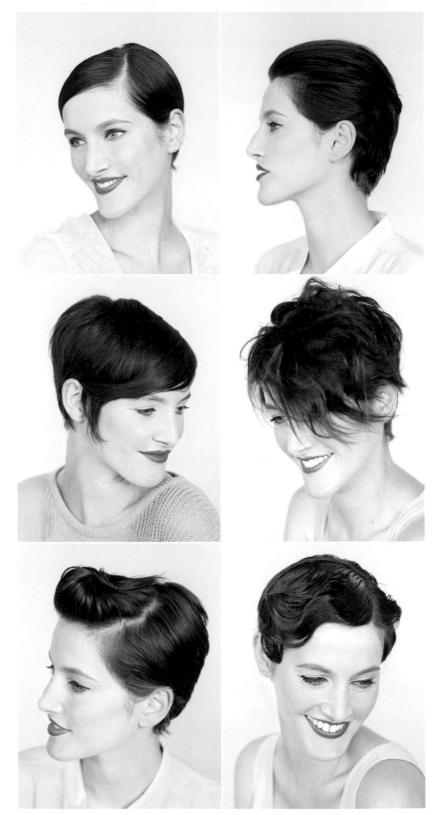

What do you mean you can't do anything with short hair? You might feel that your options are a bit more limited, but there are lots of creative styles to choose from! Plus, it's a cinch to change from style to style, so whether you want to straighten, curl, crimp, scrunch, slick forward or back or to the sides—here are six fantastic ideas for short dos!

THE SLEEK PIXIE

A cute, pert look inspired by Audrey Hepburn's iconic style.

DIFFICULTY ✂ ✂ ✂

YOU NEED
A comb, one bobby pin, hair gel

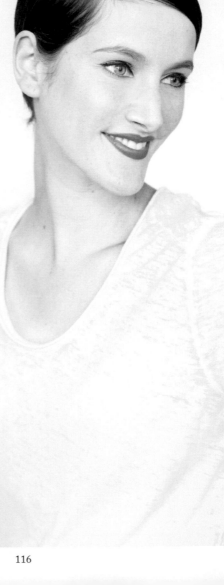

TIP
To give a boost to limp or curly hair, straighten it beforehand—makeover guaranteed!

1 Part your hair on the side.

2 Straighten out your hair with a comb.

3 Apply gel and slick the hair to the
sides using the palm of your hand.

4 Secure any excess hair behind the ear
with a bobby pin.

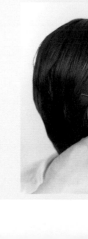

THE NEW WAVE

This ravishing minimalist do, popular with the red carpet set, will highlight your face.

DIFFICULTY ✂ ✂ ✂

YOU NEED
A comb, a brush, hair gel, styling wax

TIP
If your hair is longer at nape level, just use a small barrette in back to keep the hair together.

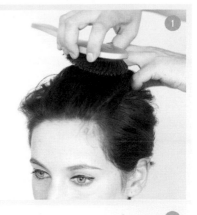

1 Brush your hair back to straighten it.

2 Apply the gel using the palm of your hand to perfectly smooth out the top of your head.

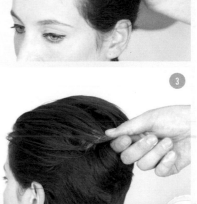

3 Massage in styling wax to bind the hair together at the back of your head.

4 Smooth all the hair back with the comb to set it firmly in place.

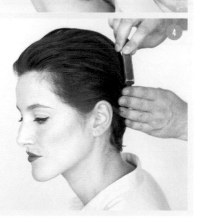

THE SIDE DO

Carefully styling one choice section of hair can change everything. This style will breathe fresh air into your usual look.

DIFFICULTY ✂ ✂ ✂

YOU NEED
A brush, one bobby pin, styling wax

TIP
Changing the side you style will change your whole look, even for mid-length hair.

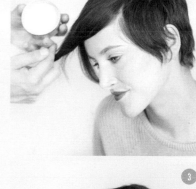

1 Brush all your hair forward in the same direction, leaving a natural part.

2 Heat up some styling wax between the palms of your hands.

3 Apply the wax all throughout the front section of hair, straightening it out.

4 Let the strands next to your ear fall toward your jaw, and pull back the front of the hair toward your ear.

5 Secure with a bobby pin.

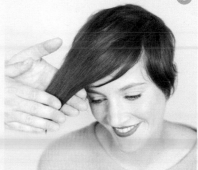

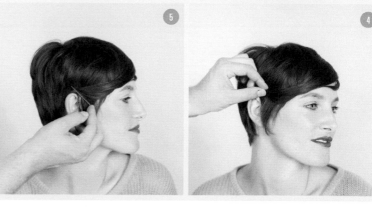

THE BEDHEAD

The striking contrast of strands sticking out and stiff ends can revive a very short cut or liven up hair that's growing back.

DIFFICULTY ✂ ✂ ✂

YOU NEED
A hair straightener, hair gel, texturizing powder

TIP

For very short hair, a hair straightener is unnecessary; the gel will be enough to straighten out the ends.

1 Tousle your hair toward the front.

2 Sprinkle texturizing powder at
the roots and work it in with your
fingers.

3 Straighten the tips of a few strands
with the hair straightener so that they
are quite stiff.

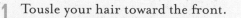

4 Set it all in place with gel.

THE PINNED-UP POUF

A subtle bouffant lock pinned over on itself makes for a refreshing yet slightly retro look.

DIFFICULTY ✂ ✂ ✂

YOU NEED
A brush, one bobby pin, hair gel

TIP
Accessorize with a headband or scarf to maximize this style's vintage potential.

1 Separate out the front section of hair and straighten it back with a brush.

2 Apply some gel using the flat of your hand.

3 Bring the hair up into a slight pouf by twisting the ends.

4 Secure at the ends using a bobby pin.

THE WAVY TWENTIES

This adorable retro hair recalls inimitable
Jazz Age style.

DIFFICULTY ✂ ✂ ✂

YOU NEED
A blow-dryer, a comb, several large
alligator clips, hair gel

TIP

*For a more modern touch, use
colored hairpins or flat barrettes
and leave them in the waves.
Besides looking sassy, it'll hold
everything in place.*

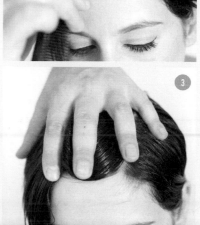

1 Part your hair on the side and apply gel throughout.

2 Trace a wave pattern with the comb.

3 Pinch the wave between your fingers, with your hand flat down, to create vertical waves as well.

4 Set the waves in place with an alligator clip, then repeat the process several times to achieve the desired effect.

5 Set it all in place by blow-drying, then gently remove the clips.

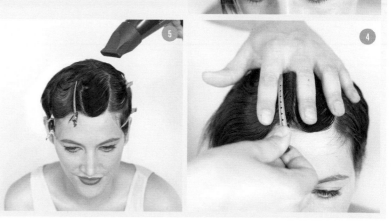

chapter 7

MID-LENGTH HAIR

in 6 styles

The Wavy Look · The Curly Bob
The Faux Bob · The Customized Half Pony
The Asymmetric Sweep · The Styled Sweep

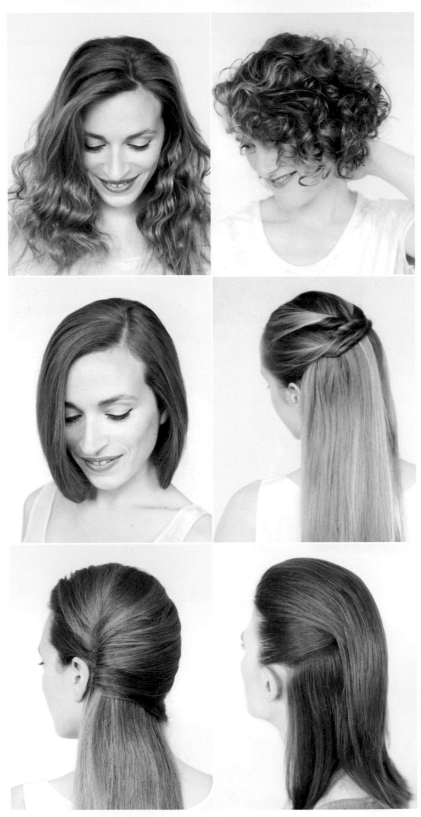

There are plenty of imaginative options for mid-length—that is, roughly down to the shoulder—hair, but the results often just fall flat. What a shame! Mid-length hair is ideal for easily maximizing volume, no-fuss straightening, or tying back in a knockout do in seconds. Make the most of it, and have fun—as you experiment, don't skimp on styling products, which can help your hair shine (and stay in place!).

THE WAVY LOOK

Gentle waves contrast naturally stiff ends in this hip, ravishing style that will instantly elevate your everyday hair.

DIFFICULTY ✂ ✂ ✂

YOU NEED
A blow-dryer, several hair elastics, texturizing saltwater spray, hair spray

TIP
Depending on how wavy you want to get, make tighter or looser braids and begin braiding closer or farther from the roots.

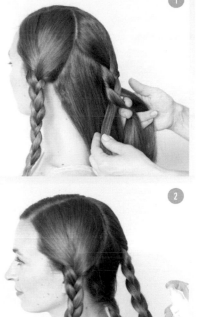

1 With damp hair, separate out several
sections of hair and braid each one,
securing each with a hair elastic
2 inches above the ends.

2 Spray texturizing saltwater spray over
the braids.

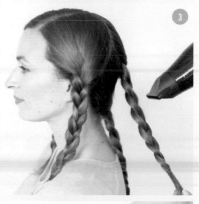

3 Blow-dry the braids.

4 Gently undo the braids and tousle
your hair with your fingers,
distributing the waves evenly over
your shoulders, then set with
hair spray.

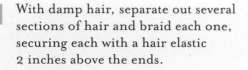

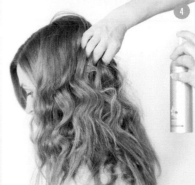

THE CURLY BOB

This nonchalant but on-trend style
is an upgrade to the classic bob.

DIFFICULTY ✂ ✂ ✂

YOU NEED
A blow-dryer, hair gel, texturizing spray,
hair spray

TIP
*You can also use spiral
curlers to get more
delicate curls.*

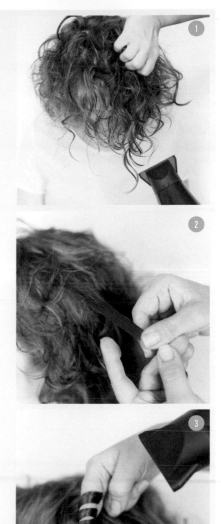

1 Pre-dry your hair top to bottom using the blow-dryer, then scrunch as you spray in texturizer to loosen up the roots.

2 On still slightly damp hair, apply gel to one small section.

3 Wrap it around a finger and dry it with the blow-dryer.

4 Repeat this process all throughout your hair, then tousle and set with hair spray.

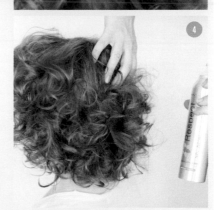

THE FAUX BOB

A clever optical illusion will give you a
striking style makeover *tout de suite*.

DIFFICULTY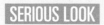

YOU NEED
A brush or a comb, one hair elastic,
fringe pins, hair spray

TIP
*For the illusion to work, the
hair at the very back needs to be
quite stiff, while the hair at the
front needs to be more soft
and flexible.*

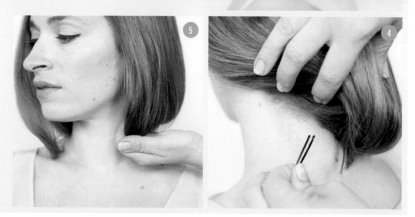

1 Part your hair on the side and carefully straighten out your hair with a comb or brush.

2 Pull your hair back into a low, looped-up ponytail secured with an elastic.

3 Turn the looped ponytail up under your hair toward the nape of your neck.

4 Secure with fringe pins at the nape.

5 Gently pull down on the hair at the sides of the "bob" to get the desired length and set with hair spray.

THE CUSTOMIZED HALF PONY

This customized version of the timeless half ponytail is ready to wear in just minutes.

DIFFICULTY ✕ ✕ ✕

YOU NEED
A brush, bobby pins, hair spray

TIP
You can make just one crisscross, if desired, or continue all the way down to your neck for a weave effect.

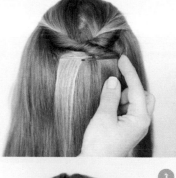

1 Pull a section of hair from the side and twist, fixing it in place with a bobby pin.

2 Repeat on the opposite side, then crisscross the two twists.

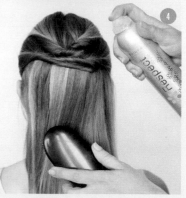

3 Repeat once again using two sections of hair a bit lower on the head, setting each crisscross parallel to the one above.

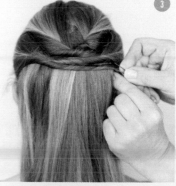

4 Brush the rest of your hair and spritz with hair spray.

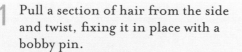

THE ASYMMETRIC SWEEP

This stunning style is classier than a ponytail, but easier than a French twist.

DIFFICULTY ⅄⅄⅄

YOU NEED
A brush, fringe pins

TIP
To achieve a bold effect, the sweep needs to be completely straight horizontally, so as to contrast with the falling vertical length of hair.

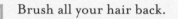

1 Brush all your hair back.

2 Sweep the hair from one side over to cover the rest of your hair.

3 Fold this sweep of hair over the rest, rolling it up inward and keeping it very firm horizontally up to ear level.

4 Secure with fringe pins, letting the remaining hair fall free.

THE STYLED SWEEP

Inspired by the catwalk, this rigid hairstyle is equal parts assertive and chic.

DIFFICULTY ✂ ✂ ✂

YOU NEED
A comb, one hair elastic, hair gel

TIP

Don't be put off by the visible effect of the gel—you need to use a lot to make the style hold. If strands persist in coming undone, just use a small bobby pin at the back.

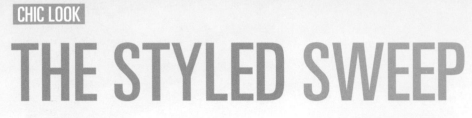

1 Separate out a section of hair the width of your forehead from the front.

2 Make a half ponytail with the sections on the side, securing with a hair elastic.

3 Smooth the sides out with gel to achieve a rigid look.

4 Fold the front section back over the elastic, lightly teasing it several times.

5 Perfectly straighten the front section with a comb and set it with gel.

chapter 8

STRAIGHT HAIR

in 6 styles

The Boosted Bun Chignon · The Bump
Beach Waves · Scrunched Ends
The Sweet Sixties · The Half Bun

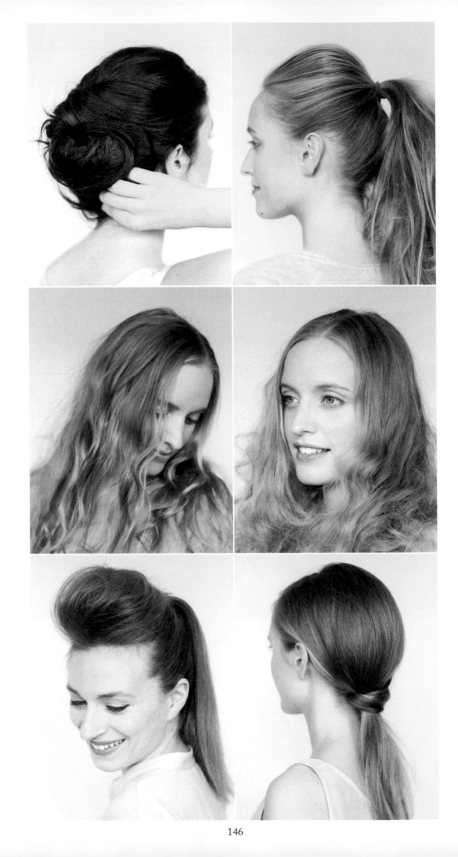

Do you ever complain that your hair is flat, thin, or impossible to style? If so, then never fear—this chapter is for you. Rest assured, flat hair is no reason to despair! All you have to do is work with it—a bit of teasing here, some texturizing products there, and before you know it, you'll be able to master styles fit for any type of hair. So enough with the drama in your morning routine. Try out these tips and styles and your relationship with your hair may just well change!

THE BOOSTED BUN CHIGNON

A bold chignon with volume
to give your hair a kick!

DIFFICULTY ✂ ✂ ✂

YOU NEED
Fringe pins, texturizing powder

TIP
*In addition to texturizing
products, you can also add volume
to a hairdo by concealing mini twists
underneath, then fluffing them up
with your fingers.*

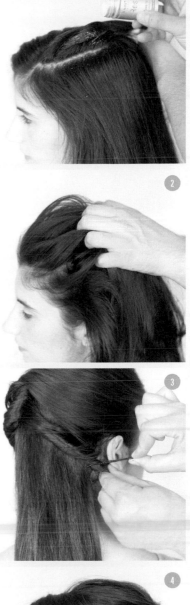

1 Apply a generous amount of
texturizing powder to your hair.

2 Scrunch your hair from the roots to
add volume as you go back.

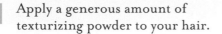

3 Take a good-sized section of hair
from one side of the forehead and
twirl it back to the opposite side,
securing it with a fringe pin. Repeat
with all remaining sections of hair
at the top, securing underneath to
thicken the mass of hair. The idea is
to create volume with twirls, which
will ultimately be hidden underneath.

4 Pull up the hair at your neck and
combine all the ends of the twirls
into a messy bun.

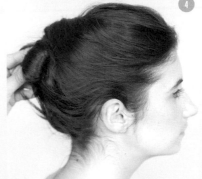

THE BUMP

The secret to this style is an accessory that bumps fine hair up into a perky curve at the top.

DIFFICULTY ✂ ✂ ✂

YOU NEED
A brush, one foam volumizing insert (or a Bumpit), one hair elastic, one large alligator clip

TIP
By placing the volumizing insert farther forward or backward, you can add volume right where you want it. Anything is possible!

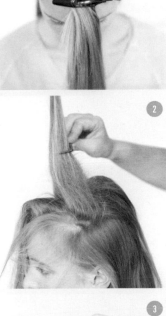

1 Separate out half your hair at the top into a half-moon and secure with the alligator clip. Then brush the hair at the back.

2 Tease the front portion of hair little by little.

3 Set the foam volumizer or Bumpit between the two sections of hair so that it stays in place.

4 Pull back the front section to cover the insert and brush back to straighten out the hair.

5 Pull all your hair together into a ponytail and secure with a hair elastic.

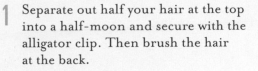

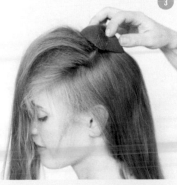

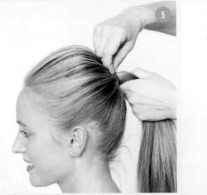

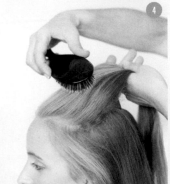

BEACH WAVES

Lightly tangled strands give this surfer-girl style a carefree, beachy look.

DIFFICULTY ⚮ ⚮ ⚮

YOU NEED
A blow-dryer, fringe pins, texturizing saltwater spray, hair spray

TIP
To modify the effect, you can vary the length of the twists or tousle at the roots.

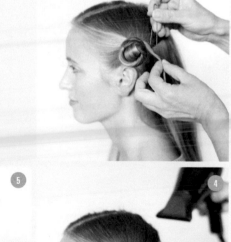

1 Apply the texturizing spray to damp hair the whole way down.

2 Take one small section and twist.

3 Twirl it up into a mini bun and secure with a fringe pin.

4 Repeat this process all around your head, then dry your hair with a blow-dryer.

5 Gently unwind the mini buns and pull on each twist to stretch it out. Tousle with your fingers and arrange to your liking, then spritz with hair spray.

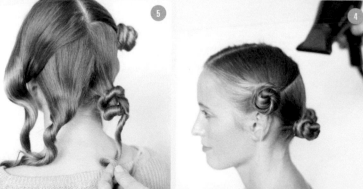

SCRUNCHED ENDS

Tasteful hints of "bed head" give a
nonchalant air to this edgy style.

DIFFICULTY ✗ ✗ ✗

YOU NEED
A brush, a blow-dryer, texturizing powder

TIP
*For more volume, finish
off teasing at the roots using
a comb, then add texturizing
powder and fluff up with
your fingers.*

1 Apply the texturizing powder to damp hair the whole way down.

2 Twist a small strand of hair, without extending all the way to the roots, and blow-dry it. Repeat with the rest of your hair.

3 Scrunch all hair.

4 Holding the brush in one hand and a section of hair in the other, tease each section, slowly moving up from ends to roots.

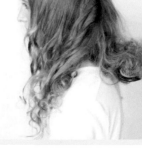

THE SWEET SIXTIES

This high bouffant is sure to bring a flirty new dimension to fine hair.

DIFFICULTY ✕ ✕ ✕

YOU NEED
A comb, one hair elastic, fringe pins

TIP
If the front part of your hair is quite long, finish off with a braid, wrapping the hair elastic inside to conceal it.

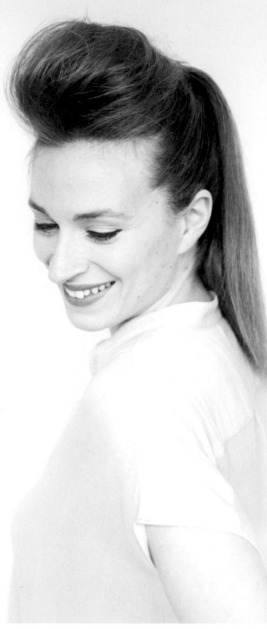

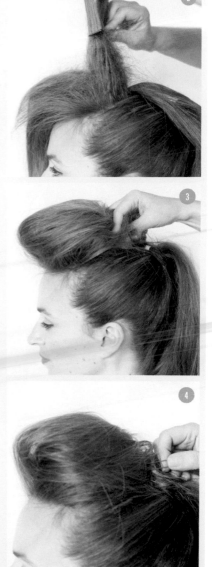

1 Separate out a triangle of hair the width of your forehead, then pull the rest back into a ponytail and secure with a hair elastic.

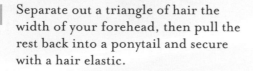

2 Use a comb to heavily tease the front section all the way from roots to ends.

3 Pull the front section back, twirling up the teased ends, then push forward to create the bouffant.

4 Secure the twirled ends with fringe pins at the same level as the ponytail elastic.

THE HALF BUN

This style combines audacious volume lift with fashionable length—a smashing look for every day.

DIFFICULTY ✗ ✗ ✗

YOU NEED
A comb, fringe pins, hair spray

TIP

This style can accommodate various lengths of hair. Try finishing off with a braid instead of a twist.

1 Part your hair on the side at the front of your head. From the back section of hair, pull out smaller sections and use a comb to tease close to the roots.

2 Flip the teased section back, then lightly smooth out the surface using a comb.

3 Bring the two front sections of hair together at the back at nape level, gently twisting them.

4 Secure the twist at the nape with fringe pins, then straighten out the remaining hair. Spritz with hair spray.

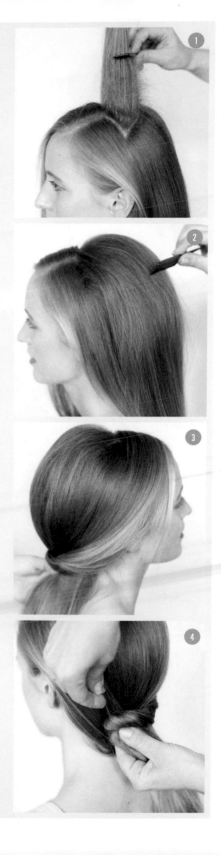

chapter 9

QUICK AND EASY

in 6 styles

The One-Shoulder · Loose Curls
The Looped-and-Low Ponytail · The Zigzag Part
Straight with a Twist · Woven Tresses

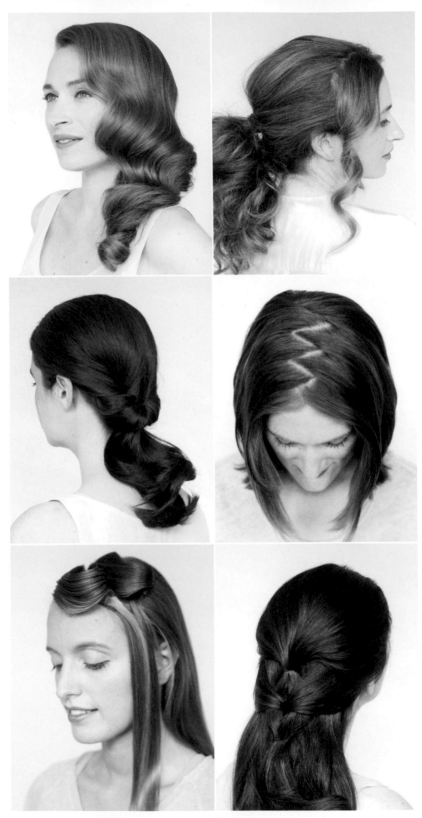

We know, we know—you don't have a personal stylist like the stars do, nor the time each morning or before a night out to make yourself look like a million bucks. But there's plenty you can do with just a little primping! Here are six ideas for super-fast and easy styles that will make it look like you spent hours prepping. Shh ... we won't tell!

THE ONE-SHOULDER

With this dramatic wavy sweep over the shoulder, you'll be ready for a night at the Oscars.

DIFFICULTY ✂ ✂ ✂

YOU NEED
A curling iron, a brush, bobby pins, smoothing serum or hair oil, hair spray

TIP
If you have curly hair, make the waves by placing hair elastics on damp hair evenly spaced out along the length.

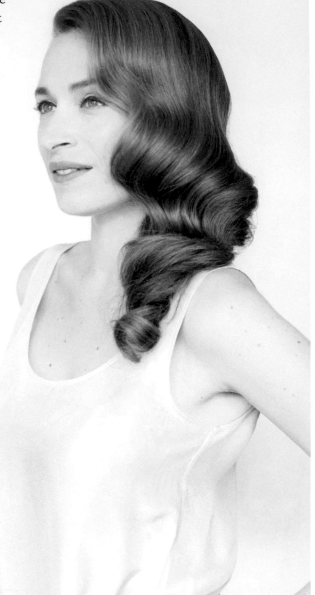

1 Use the curling iron to make corkscrew curls throughout your hair.

2 Loosen up the curls with your fingers.

3 Brush your hair flat into the palm of your hand to turn the curls into waves.

4 Smooth out the waves with smoothing serum or hair oil to help avoid static.

5 Drape your hair over one shoulder and secure in the back with a vertical line of bobby pins, then set with hair spray.

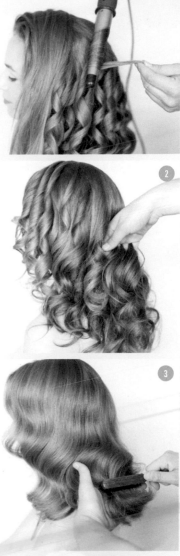

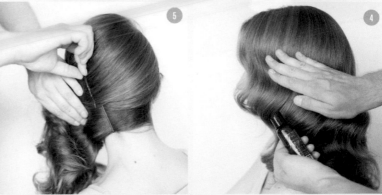

LOOSE CURLS

Low-key meets glamour in this stylish take
on the everyday ponytail.

DIFFICULTY ✂ ✂ ✂

YOU NEED
A curling iron, one hair elastic, hair spray

TIP

*If you don't have a curling
iron, you can make the curls by
twirling four or five small sections
of damp hair up into mini buns,
then blow-dry and relax
the curls.*

166

1 Use the curling iron to make fairly loose curls.

2 Tousle the curls from the top down, then spritz hair spray into the mass of hair.

3 Without pulling, gather the hair into a low ponytail and secure with an elastic, leaving several strands loose to frame your face.

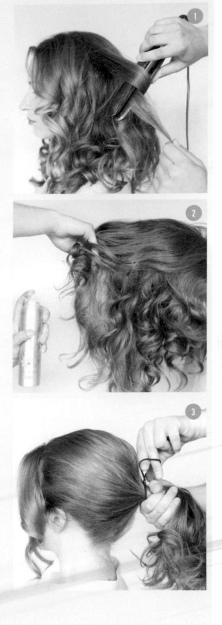

THE LOOPED-AND-LOW PONYTAIL

Upgrade your ponytail with this incredibly simple style with a classic twist.

DIFFICULTY

YOU NEED
A brush, one hair elastic

TIP
For a tighter look, repeat the process a second time or continue all the way down using multiple elastics.

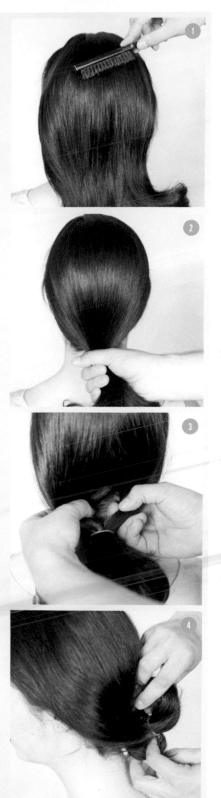

1 Brush your hair back.

2 Make a normal but low ponytail and secure with a hair elastic.

3 Make an opening just above the elastic.

4 Insert the ponytail back through the top of the opening and pull it through.

THE ZIGZAG PART

This style dresses up a center part with a jazzy angular touch—a saving grace for those morning hair emergencies!

DIFFICULTY ✂ ✂ ✂

YOU NEED
A brush, a tail comb (or use the handle of a makeup brush)

TIP
Use this method in other hairstyles to vary a side part or to create a special effect as you separate out sections of hair.

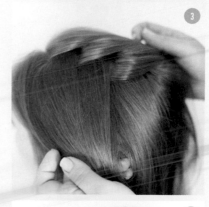

1 Comb all your hair back.

2 Place the point end of the comb vertically in the top center of your forehead, then zigzag it back without stopping.

3 Separate out the hair sections on each side to make the pattern appear.

4 Brush down your hair on each side.

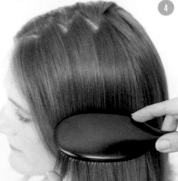

STRAIGHT WITH A TWIST

Two fanciful twists lend a dreamy look to this seductive style.

DIFFICULTY ✂ ✂ ✂

YOU NEED
Bobby pins, hair gel

TIP
If you want to conceal the ends, simply place them behind your ear.

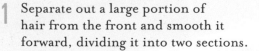

1 Separate out a large portion of hair from the front and smooth it forward, dividing it into two sections.

2 Apply gel to the rear portion and straighten it out.

3 Wrap it into a curl, then fix it to your head with a bobby pin.

4 Repeat with the second section of hair, then place next to the first curl, with the lengths of hair falling down over your cheek.

WOVEN TRESSES

Playful weaves balance out the sensible demeanor of this handsome style.

DIFFICULTY ✂ ✂ ✂

YOU NEED
A brush, three small clear elastics

TIP
For a spectacular woven effect, start this style from the forehead, or do it on both sides of your head, using small, tight weaves.

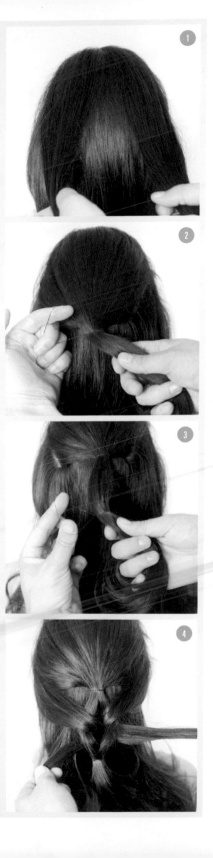

1   Brush your hair, then pull out two
sections from your temples.

2   Make these into a half ponytail,
secured with a small elastic.

3   Place a second small elastic 2 inches
below the first.

4   Separate the hair into two sections
between the two small elastics, then
pull one section of hair from each
side next to your face through this
opening. Secure these two sections
with a third small elastic, placed
about midway between the first two
elastics.

chapter 10

FOR A NIGHT OUT

in 9 styles

Victory Rolls · The Flower Pouf
The Double French Twist · The Spiral Bun
Princess Tresses · The Over-the-Head Twist
The Knotted Bun · The Hair Bow · The Half Knot

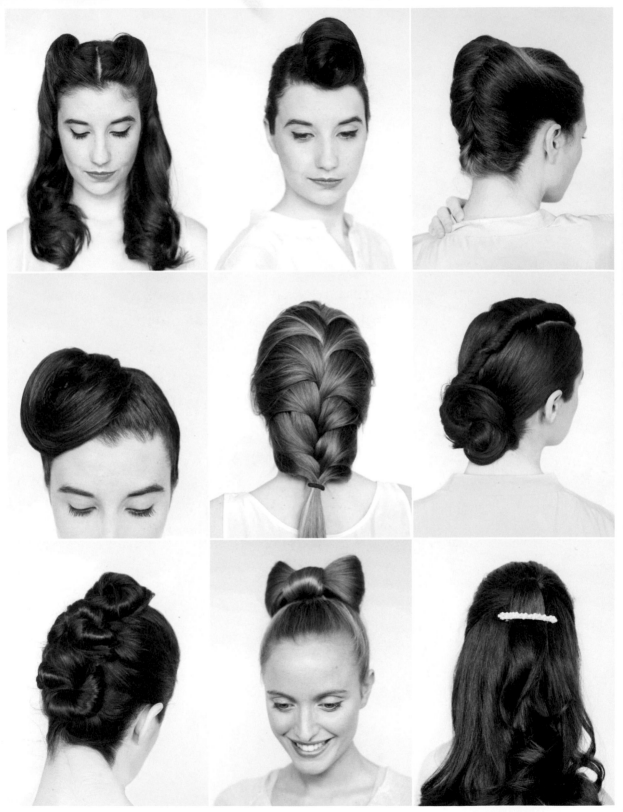

Doing your hair is often synonymous with special occasions, those times you've finally picked out your dress and shoes and all that's left is styling your hair. This chapter will help you achieve that "wow" factor for your hair as you get all dolled up for the big day—or night, as it may be. We recommend you practice the most involved styles here beforehand, but make a date of it with your girlfriends and help one another out. They'll be just as delighted as you to look dashing in a new do!

VICTORY ROLLS

This vintage look is sure to
impress and will pair well with
an art deco–style dress.

DIFFICULTY ⚔ ⚔ ⚔

YOU NEED
A comb, bobby pins, hair spray

TIP

*For the remaining hair
hanging down, feel free to
incorporate curls or pull
into a bun.*

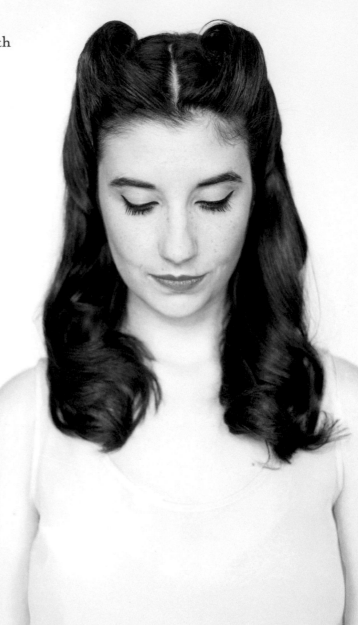

1 Divide your hair into three sections: two sections separated by a part at the top and one section at the back.

2 Take one of the front sections and tease upward.

3 Roll the section back over on itself around two fingers.

4 Secure with bobby pins, then repeat on the other side and set with hair spray.

THE FLOWER POUF

A glamorous floral twist for special occasions, this style is the ultimate accessory—pair with some simple earrings and let your hair sing.

DIFFICULTY ✂ ✂ ✂

YOU NEED
One large alligator clip, bobby pins, hair gel or hair spray

TIP

If you have trouble getting the flower to hold, wrap the hair around a small curler. This will give it the right shape while concealing the curler inside.

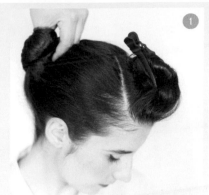

1   Separate out a wide section of hair
    at the front and secure it with an
    alligator clip, then straighten the rest
    of the hair back into a twisted bun.

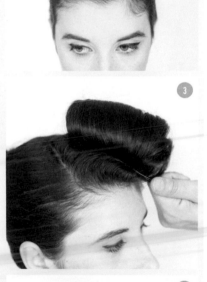

2   Carefully wrap the front section
    upward in a spiral motion.

3   Set the spiral on your head and
    secure it with bobby pins.

4   Smooth gel through the spiral to set.

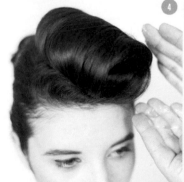

THE DOUBLE FRENCH TWIST

Here, the famous French twist gets split in two for a stunning feminine effect.

DIFFICULTY ✕ ✕ ✕

YOU NEED
A comb, bobby pins, fringe pins

TIP

For more volume, tease your hair first. If your hair slips, hide small curlers in the spirals.

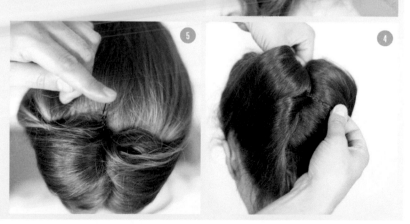

1 Take a section of hair the width of your forehead, straighten it toward the back, and secure it with bobby pins.

2 Below the bobby pins, comb to separate all the hair now at the back, creating a part.

3 Bring up the first twist, rolling the ends toward the inside and securing with fringe pins.

4 Repeat on the other side, taking care to attach the second twist to the first all along its length.

5 Stabilize the whole style by securing each twist at the top with fringe pins.

THE SPIRAL BUN

Here, the classic bun is revisited in a fabulous artistic form, perfect for galas and soirees.

DIFFICULTY ✂ ✂ ✂

YOU NEED
A brush, one hair elastic, fringe pins, wet-look gel

TIP
Vary the size of the spiral depending on the length of your hair, but make sure there's empty space in the center for visual effect.

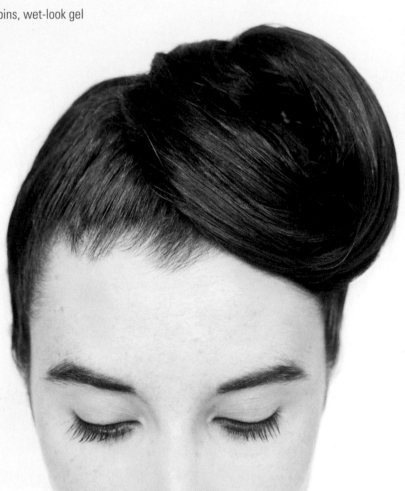

1 After brushing, make a topknot-style ponytail at the crown of your head and slightly to the side, securing with an elastic.

2 Fully coat the ponytail hair with gel and smooth out.

3 Twist the ponytail into a spiral and surround the elastic with the ends.

4 Secure the spiral with fringe pins.

PRINCESS TRESSES

This beautiful twin-weave French braid is fit for royalty.

DIFFICULTY ✕ ✕ ✕

YOU NEED
One hair elastic, hair spray

TIP
Dampen your hair to make it less slippery; this will make the process easier and help you avoid mixing up the strands.

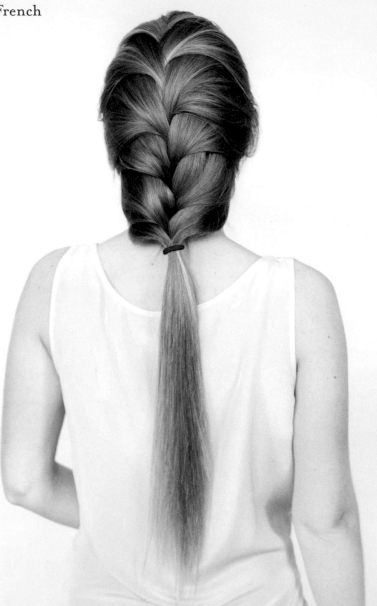

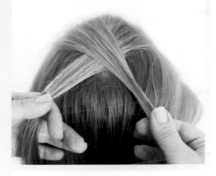

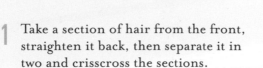

1　Take a section of hair from the front, straighten it back, then separate it in two and crisscross the sections.

2　Incorporate into each section two new sections taken from the sides and crisscrossed in turn.

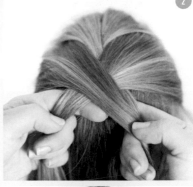

3　Continue to crisscross two sections from the outside in the same fashion, incorporating the previous weaves each time.

4　Once all side hair has been woven in, finish it off with the hair elastic and set with hair spray.

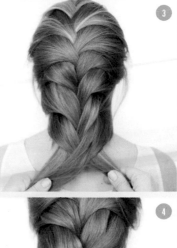

THE OVER-THE-HEAD TWIST

You'll be ready for the catwalk with this supremely stylish chignon, almost a haute couture accessory in itself.

DIFFICULTY ✂ ✂ ✂

YOU NEED
Fringe pins, hair spray, hair gel
or straightening spray

TIP
*If your hair is very long,
slip the bun into a discreet
hairnet, which will help set it
more easily.*

1 Divide your hair into two sections:
a large rectangle starting from the
forehead and including the crown,
and then the rest of your hair.

2 Pull the back section of your hair so
that it is perfectly straight, using the
straightening spray or hair gel, and
secure it in a low bun or ponytail.

3 Pull the top section of your hair into
a tight twist, rolling it over on itself
toward the back like a small roller,
following one of the part lines.

4 Attach the twist to the bun with fringe
pins and set with hair spray.

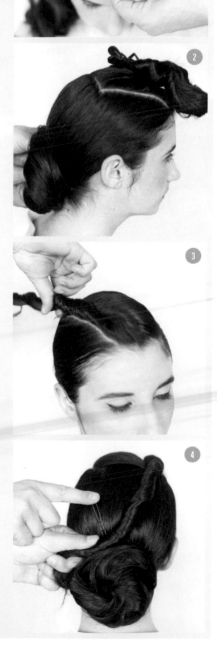

THE KNOTTED BUN

An intricate triple-tiered bun to adorn
all hair types.

DIFFICULTY ✗ ✗ ✗

YOU NEED
Several small clear elastics, fringe pins,
hair spray

TIP
*If your hair is dull
or rough, apply hair oil to
add some shine.*

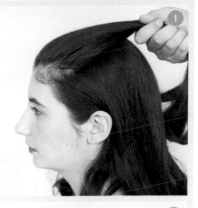

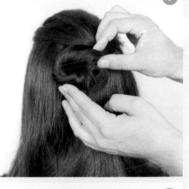

1 Pull back the hair from the front third of your head into a ponytail and secure with a small elastic.

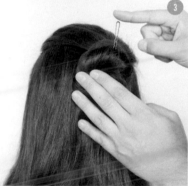

2 Twist the ponytail, then wrap it around itself to form a bun.

3 Secure the bun with fringe pins.

4 Repeat two or three times, depending on how much hair is left, taking care to align all buns vertically. Set with hair spray.

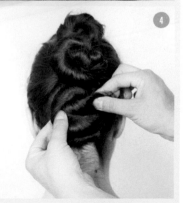

THE HAIR BOW

This imaginative style is always a knockout hit—little do others know just how simple the style is to create!

DIFFICULTY ✕ ✕ ✕

YOU NEED
One hair elastic, fringe pins

TIP
For the bow to hold up, the initial loop can't be too wide; otherwise, the sides will be limp and the bow will droop.

1 Pull your hair up into a folded
ponytail high on your head, the ends
falling far forward.

2 Separate the ponytail hair into two
sections.

3 Pass the end of the ponytail over the
middle of the divided hair, making
sure it is smooth and straight.

4 Secure the end behind the bow
with fringe pins and conceal the
remaining hair under the bow
around the elastic.

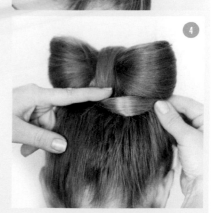

THE HALF KNOT

This refined style is ideal for special occasions, but will take no time to whip up.

DIFFICULTY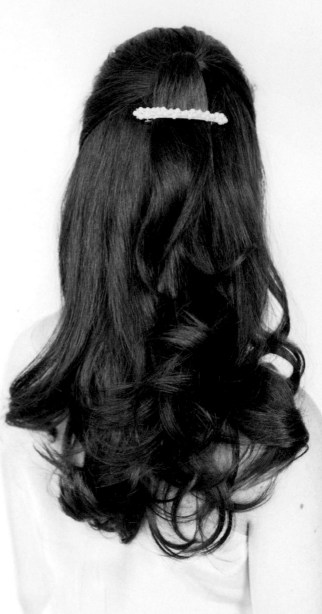

YOU NEED
A brush, a wide barrette, hair spray

TIP
To achieve a clean look, don't ease up on the tension: keep the hair firmly grasped in your hands until you attach the barrette.

1 Brush your hair thoroughly and divide the front part into two smooth, straight sections.

2 Pull the hair back and knot the two sections without releasing the tension.

3 Pivot the hair vertically.

4 Flip the top portion down over the bow and fix it in place with a barrette. Spritz with hair spray.

GLOSSARY

STYLING TOOLS

ALLIGATOR CLIP

This versatile clip has two flat lips that come together to hold hair in place. Perfect for setting a style or for holding hair in place while you work another part of your hair. This clip doesn't have any teeth, so it won't leave any bumps in your hair when you remove it.

BOBBY PINS

One of the most basic styling tools, bobby pins are flat metal hairpins used to pinch together small sections of hair. An essential for updos, but useful for many styles.

CURLER OR ROLLER

Perhaps outdated as a means of curling your hair, curlers are still useful, especially for hiding inside certain hairdos to add volume or provide stability.

CURLING IRON

A long, wand-shaped heating device used to heat-set curls of various sizes. Choose between models with a clamp or newer, conical versions without a clamp.

FRINGE PINS

Similar to bobby pins, fringe pins are U-shaped, with more space between the prongs, and give a less tight hold. Perfect for holding sections of hair together and setting styles in place.

HAIR DONUT OR DONUT RING

A ring-shaped accessory usually made of foam, through which hair can be pulled and set into a bun. Especially useful for large-volume buns.

HAIR ELASTIC

The standard hair tie, made of fabric-covered elastic, used to hold hair back, especially in ponytails.

HAIR STRAIGHTENER OR FLAT IRON

An elongated, clamplike device with two heated ceramic plates used for straightening hair or creating waves. Some newer all-in-one versions offer both straightening and curling capabilities.

HAIR VOLUMIZER OR BUMPIT

A bulging, rounded accessory made of foam or plastic, concealed inside certain hairdos to add volume and shape. You may recognize these as "Bumpits" from infomercials.

SMALL CLEAR ELASTIC

Small, usually transparent elastics made of plastic, used to hold back hair or to secure braids and twists. Clear versions are popular since they don't stand out, but colored elastics are available too.

SPIRAL CURLERS OR ROLLERS

Narrow, pliable tubes made of flexible plastic that can be adjusted to your desired shape, around which locks of hair can be wound to form tight curls.

STYLING PRODUCTS

HAIR GEL

Gel fixes hair in place by adhering strands together. Also referred to as fixing gel or styling gel.

HAIR SPRAY

The classic fixing spray, hair spray holds hair in place from the outer surface.

SALTWATER SPRAY

Saltwater spray, a relatively new texturizing option, is used to achieve a rough look, as if you've just gone for a dip in the ocean, and is especially useful for bohemian styles. It also helps slick hair cling better.

SMOOTHING SERUM

An essential product for thick, curly hair, smoothing serum softens the hair and makes brushing easy.

STRAIGHTENING CREAM

This cream is ideal for smoothing long and fine hair and preventing frizz.

STRAIGHTENING SPRAY

This spray protects hair from the heat of a flat iron or hairdryer while sealing in smoothness to extend the life of a straight do.

TEXTURIZING POWDER

A secret of the pros, texturizing powder has thickening and fixing properties to help transform smooth, slick, or unruly hair into stable, easy-to-work hair that can withstand any style.

TEXTURIZING SPRAY

Texturizing spray lightly fixes hair, thickens, and adds volume.

WAX

Hair wax, or styling wax, is worked deep into hair usually after being heated up by rubbing between your fingers or hands. Waxes come in varying thickness and stickiness, depending on whether for use in texturizing or fixing hair in place. Ideal for short hair.

WET-LOOK GEL

A looser gel than standard styling gel, wet-look gel smoothes out hair and gives it a shiny, almost wet look.

TECHNIQUES

SCRUNCHING

Scrunching involves fluffing up or aerating your hair, using your fingers to add volume and shape. Should be accompanied by a texturizing product.

SLICKING

Slicking hair involves smoothing out a section of hair to reduce volume and achieve a visible sleek effect.

STRAIGHTENING

Straightening, using either a brush or hair product, flattens hair and removes volume and curls.

TEASING OR BACKCOMBING

Teasing, in which hair is combed in the opposite direction as you normally would—in the direction of the roots rather than toward the ends—creates volume. Either a comb or brush can be used.

WAVES

A natural-seeming wavy look can be achieved by loosening up curls made with a curling iron, or by undoing small buns or twists of hair that have been set, then blow-dried.

INDEX OF STYLES

BUNS

EASY BUNS

BRAIDED BUNS

CLASSY BUNS

BRAIDS

BASIC BRAIDS

HEADBANDS

ACCESSORIES

CURLY, WAVY, AND KINKY HAIR

SHORT HAIR

MID-LENGTH HAIR

STRAIGHT HAIR

QUICK AND EASY

FOR A NIGHT OUT

Additional Acknowledgments

A huge thank-you to the staffs at Provalliance and Saint Algue—Amélie, Lor, Olivia Provost, Claire Dubuit, Gwenola Ferrien, and Margaux Cabaussel—for their invaluable help and enthusiasm for the project. Also many thanks to the expert stylists who guided me along.

Thanks to stylists William Cerf, Gaétan Guégan, and Carole Le Bris for their skill, sure-handedness, and helpful hints.

Thanks to Brigitte for her sense of humor, kindness, and sharp set of eyes, as well as for her priceless assistant, Blue.

Thanks to Anne Rabasse, Lori Beraisina, Margaux Held, Marie-Amélie Lebeau, Olivia Maschio Esposito, Pauline Renier, and Solène Duclos for posing as models.

Thanks to Justine, from American Vintage Passy, in Paris, for her wise advice.

And thank you, readers and friends, for sharing your suggestions, as well as your hair emergencies, all of which were an endless source of inspiration as I looked for fun, creative new ways for us to style our hair.